The Black Woman's

BEAUTY BOOK

*A complete guide to great looks
with advice from top experts
on hair, skin, and makeup*

· — · — · — · — · — · — · — · — · — · — · — · — · — · — · — · — ·

*Illustrations by Catherine Clayton Purnell
Photographs by Barbara DuMetz
Hair and makeup by Stanley James*

The Black Woman's

BEAUTY BOOK

* * * * * * * * * * * * * *

La Verne Powlis

DOUBLEDAY & COMPANY, INC.   GARDEN CITY, NEW YORK

Library of Congress Cataloging in Publication Data
Powlis, La Verne, 1947–
    The Black woman's beauty book.

    1. Beauty, Personal.   2. Women, Black—Health and hygiene.   I. Title.
RA778.P883   646.7′2′024042
ISBN: 0-385-14450-4
Library of Congress Catalog Card Number 78–22349
9 8 7 6 5 4 3

*To my wonderful father who instilled in me the
sweet taste of independence when he taught me how
to braid my own hair.*

*To my mother who ushered me into her world of
beauty by surrounding me with perfumes, powders,
creams . . . and love.*

ACKNOWLEDGMENTS My experiences while writing this book are among my most treasured because of the special people who contributed so much to me along the way. I would like to pause and say a humble thank-you to:

An incredible team, Catherine, Barbara, and Stanley, the best who consistently gave their best, and to Leslie Smith whose assistance helped me complete the manuscript in half the time.

The dermatologists in the National Medical Association for their willingness to share their very special knowledge. Especially to Dr. John A. Kenney, Jr., and Dr. Harold Pierce for their review of the manuscript.

To Lydia Sarfati at Klisar and Louis Modica at the Louis M Salon and their staffs, especially to Bruce Clark who introduced me to all the right people.

The women who graciously sat to have their hair cut, styled, their makeup done, then sat in front of the camera without air conditioning during those hot summer days in July—Olga Adderley, Sheila Anderson, Margaret Calhoun, Madeline Cleare, Sylvia Davis, Esther Downing, Arlene Fridie, Juliette Gore, Connie Stewart, Brenda Williams.

To my very first editor, Arthur Hettich at *Family Circle* magazine, who gave a young Black writer a chance.

All the editors at *Bride's* magazine and Vickie Peslak for her help in poring through hundreds of slides. Especially to my editor-in-chief, Barbara Tober, for her unrelenting encouragement and support.

To my friends, many who read the manuscript in various stages, others for just being there: Linda Dannenberg, Esther Downing, Delores and Karl Friedman, Anita Gates, Nell and Bert Gibson, Violet Hazael, Joe Hickman, Raeanne Hytone, Joyce Kuykendall, Byron Lewis, Charlotte Lipson, Cindy Morris, Carlos Overr, Pepta Pierre, Alberta Russell, Connie Stewart, and my sister, La Von.

Sherry Knox, my editor, who instinctively believed in an idea whose time had come, and Carol Mann, my agent, for being the catalyst that made it all happen.

Most of all, to my family and church whose prayers sustained me through it all.

CONTENTS

• - •

• - • - • - • - • - • - • - • ·HAIR CARE· • - • - • - • - •

⸺STYLING AND TREATMENTS⸺

·········SKIN CARE·········

MAKEUP

·······IMAGE·······

·······A CLOSING NOTE·······

The Black Woman's

BEAUTY BOOK

INTRODUCTION The billion-dollar cosmetics industry, which develops hundreds of new products every season, has created an insatiable demand for beauty information. National women's magazines and specialty beauty books are designed to meet this need, but, with a few exceptions, this information is primarily geared to the white consumer. You, the Black woman, who spends a greater portion of your disposable income on beauty products, have been largely forgotten.

This is probably because cosmetics for us were generally unavailable until the past decade or so, when black cosmetic companies led the way in marketing products complementary to our hair and skin. Gradually their profitable success inspired the international cosmetic giants to enter this lucrative segment of the beauty market. Today, the results across the board are updated research, new product development, and greater availability of quality cosmetics that offer Black women their money's worth.

Somewhere along the way, though, a gap had inadvertently occurred. Beauty products designed especially for us were now available. But sufficient, generic information on how to select and use these products was still missing.

As a beauty and health editor, I was particularly aware of this gap. I realized the wealth of information available to us and became increasingly concerned with the need to put it all together. Therefore I have researched, compiled, translated, and finally written this beauty information to answer your questions—and mine.

I began my research with Black dermatologists—doctors specifically skilled in the care and treatment of our hair, skin, and nails. The views and information from this highly specialized group are represented throughout this book in an effort to present you with the facts. I incorporate dermatological information as it relates to health and beauty.

Once I digested the medical facts, I expanded my research to include hair-care specialists, hairstylists, skin-care experts, and makeup artists. Basic fashion tips from leading pros complete your beauty image. All of these experts, top in their fields, work with some of the world's most beautiful women—models, singers, actresses—and between these pages they share their seasoned tricks-of-the-trade with you.

I've also included material from seminars, conferences, and courses that I've attended throughout my years in the beauty field. Together with my own knowledge as an editor, I present it all to you in *The Black Woman's Beauty Book.*

The tips and advice in this first comprehensive handbook are tailored to help you save money by offering you guidelines in selecting the right products, while minimizing your salon visits. As such, it is a reference book, to be read through completely, then consulted time and again, year after year.

This is basically a how-to book, both how-to-do and how-to-know. It is for you, today's Black woman, who enjoys the unique luxury of being beautiful on your own terms. I sincerely hope you enjoy reading it. Most of all, I trust that it will help you to excerise all of your beauty options and to discover the incredible woman you really are. Because when a Black woman is beautiful, she's like nothing else the world has ever seen.

For Starters: Diet and Exercise

I strongly subscribe to the standard beauty trinity of proper rest, at least eight hours of sleep; a well-balanced diet, with a concentration of fresh fruits, vegetables, and fish; and exercise, whether it's dance, sports, or martial arts.

COPPER CUNNINGHAM/ACTRESS, MODEL

Good beauty habits should begin when you're a teenager and follow you into adulthood. Feed your skin properly, beginning with the right vitamins. Avoid junk foods. Your skin and teeth pay if you drink lots of sweets and sodas. When you're thirsty, think in terms of fresh water, which naturally flushes your system.

MARCIA MCBROOM/ACTRESS, MODEL

Exercises like yoga and running put me in a better
space, especially when I don't feel happy or up to par.
The benefits are not only external, but internal.
My mind relaxes while my body gets released.
Every once in a while I eliminate poisons from my
system by fasting for a couple of days. It helps me
feel lighter, clearer, and, at my age, helps my bones
to feel better.

OLGA ADDERLEY/ACTRESS
(photo right)

I believe in body consciousness, that you can
determine how strong your body will be, how it
will look. You can develop a great body, just give it
a little attention a few minutes every day. Jogging
is very good for your body, face, and skin. It tones
the muscles, improves circulation, and develops
discipline—all have a positive effect on the total you.
Alternate your exercise by jumping rope twenty
minutes a day, three times a week. To keep your body
in control, constantly think about it. Tighten the
muscles in your stomach and buttocks, correct your
posture, straighten your shoulders, and walk tall.

BETHANN HARDISON/RUNWAY MODEL

For these successful Black models and actresses, diet and exercise overwhelmingly form the basis of a lifetime beauty regimen that makes them look and feel good every day. These women illustrate that the fundamental secrets of beauty are not so complex after all.

How well you nourish and take care of your body reflects itself in the healthiness of your hair and nails, the flawlessness of your skin, your body weight and structure, and your overall sense of well-being. When you begin by taking care of you from the *inside,* you are giving yourself the best you have, and it will be reflected naturally, and beautifully, on the *outside.*

YOU ARE WHAT YOU EAT What your body feeds upon is one of the most important factors that determines how beautiful you will feel. And feeling beautiful is 90 per cent of being beautiful. Exercising all of your beauty potential means having an operating consciousness of which foods turn your body on and which ones slow it down.

Supplying yourself with the essential foods, such as a balanced amount of protein (meat, fish, eggs), carbohydrates (sugar and starches), fat, fiber, vitamins, and minerals, means that life-sustaining nutrients are being absorbed into the bloodstream where they are further transmitted to the cells that feed your skin, hair, and nails. For this reason, the effectiveness of hair foods and vitamins that "make hair grow" is questionable, because if you are eating the right foods, you are already getting your daily requirements. Just remember to take care of your body and it will take care of you.

FRESH IS BEST In most cases, fresh, natural products are best for you. We've heard a thousand times before that too much sugar causes obesity, diabetes, tooth decay, coronary ailments, and bowel problems. What we should also realize is that many foods contain hidden sugars, and examples are soft drinks, pastries, and many prepared foods.

We are also aware of the importance of limiting the amount of fat and cholesterol in our diets. We know that an excessive intake of salt may cause high blood pressure, acid retention in the stomach, and stomach cancer. But overuse also contributes significantly to those minor irritations like premenstrual swelling, cramps, and headaches.

If you're on a low-sodium diet, remember that some vegetables, peanut butter, breads, milk, cheese, eggs, and alcoholic beverages are high in sodium content.

Caffeine in tea, cocoa, soda, aspirins, antihistamines, and coffee stimulates the heart and also causes gastric secretions in the system. Too much caffeine could result in restlessness, anxiety, low blood sugar, diarrhea, stomach ulcers, glaucoma, and heart disease.

If you must have coffee, decaffeinated is better, or try to substitute with natural herb teas altogether, which is your best alternative and a delicious one, too.

FOOD ALLERGIES So often we accept feeling bad, not quite like ourselves, as a common course of life when, in fact, it is not. If we listen to our body, it will help us to help ourselves. When it signals depression and fatigue, then you cannot look your best because you certainly are not feeling your best.

What is an allergy? It's a reaction to a substance that is different from most other people's reactions. Some individuals have bad reactions to certain foods; others do not. This is what is called "biochemic individuality" and means that what may be great for someone else may give you an adverse reaction.

In many tests involving Black, Indian, and Asian children, it was found that drinking milk caused hostility, sleepiness, and confusion in the children. Much of the disturbance in classrooms was eliminated when milk was omitted from the breakfast menu. This means that for many of us, milk can often cause an allergic reaction evidenced as either stomach cramps and/or irritability. Again, your tolerance for milk depends on your own biochemic individuality.

Of vital importance is the realization that symptoms such as depression, anger, anxiety, fatigue, feeling fuzzy-headed, loss of memory, headaches, and skin disorders frequently indicate an allergic reaction to certain foods. Often it's not the food group itself that is harmful but the chemical processes it has been put through, like those used to preserve beef to make it cosmetically appealing.

Foods that have lots of preservatives, artificial coloring, flavor enhancers, thickeners, and bleaches contain chemicals that are primary sources of food allergies.

YOUR AT-HOME ALLERGY TEST   If you feel sluggish and irritable shortly after a meal, think about what you ate. If you suspect a certain food as being the culprit (sugar, wheat, beef, cheese), eliminate that food from your diet completely for a week or two. In many cases you get a good result if you fast completely for four to five days during the time you are testing yourself for a food allergy, but this should only be done under your doctor's supervision.

After your system has been sufficiently cleared of this food, try it again and see if you get another bad reaction. If you do, you are allergic to this food and should check labels carefully for other foods that may contain this ingredient.

Often, how your food is packaged can also affect you. Plastic, for instance, is high on the list of materials that cause adverse reactions, and if you drink water bottled in plastic and constantly have headaches, the plastic absorbed into the water may be causing the problem.

Food allergies can be aggravated by mental stress and tension, as well as vitamin and mineral deficiencies. So analyze your entire diet and be objective about your state of mind before you panic. If you suspect that what you are eating is making you feel ill, then seek the help of a qualified nutritionist and have your diet analyzed.

You may even need to undergo a series of food-allergy tests, but this can be expensive and is only advised if your problem is severe. You may like to read some of the very outstanding books available on the subject of food allergies, excessive salt and sugar in the American diet, and the benefits of fasting, to help you tune in to your own body's needs.

EXERCISE IS GOOD FOR YOUR HEAD   Daily exercise is a large part of the priority list for good health and beauty. Dull and lifeless hair and skin can very well be the extension of a dull and lifeless body.

There is a category of exercises coined "aerobics," by its father, Kenneth H. Cooper, M.D., M.P.H., that are particularly excellent for both mind and body. In fact, these exercises are part of the official Air Force exercise program.

Basically, aerobic exercises involve your entire system and provide life-lengthening stimulation for your heart and lungs, sending fresh blood pumping throughout your body, right to the very top of your head. Brisk walking, running, jumping rope, swimming, bicycling, dancing, tennis, and racket ball are daily exercises that are great for overall well-being.

The most popular of these aerobics is running, and here are what I feel are the main reasons why: Primarily, it is fun and exhilarating. It takes you outside, away from those four walls, placing you in direct contact with nature. You don't have to attend any class in order to begin, or wait for someone to run with you, or for any particular time of day. You run when the spirit moves you, for as long as you want to, where you want to. It's inexpensive. Your main investment is a good pair of running sneakers and it might be a good idea to get them a half-size larger, to make room for thick socks.

Running is one of the best ways to firm up those buttocks, hips, and thighs—areas where nature has been particularly gracious to us. It also strengthens the arms, firms breasts and tummy. Always wear a bra or close-fitting swimsuit when running. Don't wear makeup; the open pores will absorb it. Apply a moisturizer if you run in cool weather; when the air quality is not good, try to alternate running with an indoor activity like jumping rope.

And before you run that first block, be sure to have a thorough checkup and begin *only* with your doctor's authorization.

WARMING UP　No matter what your choice for exercise, remember, don't overdo it. Always warm up with jumping jacks, sit-ups, deep knee bends, and stretching, to prepare your body before beginning your exercise. Fifteen to twenty minutes are considered a good amount of warm-up time.

Start slowly at first, breathing deeply as you exercise. If you are running, you should be able to talk *while* you are running. If you can't, you are probably running too fast.

If your body screams "hurt" or "tired," slow down gradually and walk until your pulse rate returns to normal. If you are still perspiring, that's an indication that you have not cooled down sufficiently. Keep moving until you do.

If you are just beginning your aerobic exercise routine, this chart from *Bride's* magazine will help you decide which exercise is good for you, depending on the amount of time you have available. Don't be discouraged if you don't feel like swimming or running every day. Four days out of seven are a good minimum. What's important is that you enjoy your exercise and that will help you to be fairly consistent.

HOW MUCH EXERCISE DO YOU NEED?

	EVERY DAY	FIRST TIME
SWIMMING	½ mile or 30 minutes	15 minutes; take it easy
JOGGING	2–2½ miles or 20 minutes	10 minutes; alternate jogging, walking
TENNIS	25–30 minutes, normal game	15 minutes, normal game
BIKING	2–3 miles, easy speed	10–15 minutes, easy speed
WALKING	1–1½ miles in 10–20 minutes (brisk)	15–20 minutes, avoid hills

THIS CHART SPECIALLY PREPARED FOR *BRIDE'S* BY THE YWCA OF NEW YORK CITY
Copyright © 1978 by the Condé Nast Publications, Inc.

Now that you've laid the groundwork for getting your body to feel good from the inside out, let's consider what your beauty options are for your hair, your skin, and your makeup.

Hair
Care

Hair, the Natural Adornment

• •

Hair is the body's natural adornment. Keeping it healthy and beautiful means grooming our hair so that it maintains its natural texture, is manageable and easy to style.

The more familiar we become with understanding our hair's texture, the more we realize that several options are ours when we style our hair. We can decide to release our hair's curliness a little or a lot. Or we can decide not to alter our hair's character at all. With today's new aesthetic, we celebrate our texture.

In this new school of hair-care philosophy, the less you have to do to your hair, the more it functions for you, today's active Black woman. Less does not mean neglect, but rather a routine that has been streamlined to allow you more freedom.

And fun! Your hair can and should be fun to work with, never a chore or a bother. These chapters will help you discover your real beauty potential. Dermatologists and beauty experts pioneering in the field of Black hair care share their techniques, treatments, and information to help you have the loveliest hair possible.

You will find specifics on how to choose products, the correct way to shampoo and set your hair, and which kinds of haircuts flatter your face shape. Step-by-step instructions for relaxing your hair at home are included, along with the new technique for thermal pressing called défrisage. For the natural wearer, you will learn how to trim your Afro at home, plus how to style it so that you can get three different looks.

You may be surprised to find that treatments and styles you thought you had to avoid are now adaptable to your hair, and that hair-care habits you've had for years may be doing more harm than good. Quick, easy techniques free you from elaborate, old-fashioned, time-consuming treatments.

Now learn how simple it is to have hair that looks and feels *beautiful*.

You Deserve the Best

If something is really worth having, you can be sure there's a price tag attached. The investment can be time, patience, or money, and all too often, it's all three. One thing is for sure—the best things in life are *not* free.

This is especially true when it comes to caring for your hair. You need, and your hair deserves, the skilled expertise only a professional can offer. It's the only way you can get individualized hair care designed for your particular needs.

Visiting a salon regularly is not a luxury, it's a necessity, your investment toward having lovely, healthy hair. How you handle your hair at home is equally important and the trained stylist can educate and guide you by making suggestions and offering cautions.

TEAMWORK   You and your stylist should work together as a team, consulting with each other, educating each other about how your hair reacts to new products and treatments. Your hairstylist should be someone you have the utmost confidence in, someone who listens to you and works with you in developing your hair's fullest beauty potential. And it doesn't matter whether your hair is natural, relaxed, or défrisaged, the requirements are the same for trimming, conditioning, and care.

CHOOSING A SALON   Because of the expense and varying qualities of expertise, you should be as careful in choosing your salon as you are in selecting a doctor. You are making the investment of your time and beauty dollar, and you deserve the absolute best.

If there are many salons in your area, deciding on which salon to go to can be confusing. However, a beautiful head is the best advertisement. Stop women you see, whose hair you admire, and ask them about their salon.

Your first visit to a new salon should be just for consultation. It's always best to call for an appointment and to specify that this will be your first visit.

Choosing a salon begins the minute you pick up the phone. Is the receptionist polite, helpful, courteous? There is no charge for consultation, and if you are told the salon is too busy to discuss your hair needs with you, then they obviously already have all the clients they can accommodate.

A half hour is adequate time for you to ask questions and to let the stylist examine your hair. Expect him to ask you questions, too. When was the last time you had your hair cut and by whom? What kind of shampoo, relaxer, conditioning treatments have you received? How often do you shampoo at home? What kind of rollers do you use? Is the style you are wearing your usual preference? Then and only then, when your stylist has taken the time to find about your hair's history, is he or she equipped to make recommendations as to what is best for you.

Feel free to ask your stylist what products and treatments will be used on your hair. It's your right to know. If you travel frequently, you want to be able to make suggestions to any new salon you may visit, or know what to purchase to care for your hair yourself.

During your consultation, be aware of the way the other patrons are treated. Do you like the looks of their hair? Are the styles contemporary? Do you like the *ambiance* of the salon? Is it clean, well lighted, airy, cheerful? Feeling comfortable and relaxed are, after all, a large part of the services you are paying for. Keep searching for the right salon until you are satisfied.

BY APPOINTMENT ONLY Time is money, and the fast pace of the American lifestyle demands prompt service and appointments that are honored. This also means that you have to hold up your end of the responsibility by making appointments well in advance and canceling, if necessary, well in advance, too.

Making an appointment is not an added service, something for which you should be charged extra. It's part of your beauty dollar, and if yours is a busy schedule, you want to know that you can get in and out of the salon within a reasonable amount of time.

THE ETIQUETTE OF TIPPING Tipping is your way of saying that you are pleased with how you look. Generally, your tip should be approximately 15 per cent of your total bill. This means that if you have one person wash your hair, another set it, another cut and style it, you divide the total amount of your tip among all three, with the largest portion going to the person who cut and styled your hair. *Example:* $35 total bill—$1.00 for wash, $1.00 for set, $3.00 for cut and style.

If your hairstylist has done you a favor by giving you a last-minute appointment, or cutting your hair when you weren't scheduled for a cut, show your appreciation by tipping a little extra. It is not necessary ever to tip the proprietor of a salon, even though he or she may have personally styled your hair.

Tip your manicurist separately, but be sure to deduct the amount of your manicure from the total amount of your bill in figuring out the remainder of your tips.

TRIM IT Usually, a good rule of thumb is to visit your salon at least once a month—the absolute minimum. Your hairstylist can alert you to problems like split ends and breakage early. Don't wait until your hair's condition is so severe that what you really need is a magic wand instead of a hair comb. Miracles come from heaven; they do not occur in the stylist's chair.

Hair that is in good condition need only be trimmed once every three or four months. You should get a good deep-conditioning treatment at least once or twice a month.

With this kind of care and attention, supplemented by a sensible home hair-care routine, your hair has the opportunity to look its best. And when your hair looks good, you have that extra little bounce in your step and added confidence that says you have a slight edge on the world.

The Right Care for Delicate Hair

· ·

The fragile, delicate nature of our hair demands treatments and products that are specifically designed for Black women. Primarily, however, the way we handle our hair at home between salon visits determines how healthy our hair will be.

Without realizing it, we can sometimes put undue stress on our hair, inadvertently causing painful, temporary or even permanent, hair loss. By painful, I mean that heartbreak you experience when your hair is breaking and you can't quite figure out why. First, let's distinguish between this and normal hair growth and loss.

ANATOMY OF A HAIR   Hair is actually an extension of the skin, and one of its purposes is to protect and regulate body temperature. Each hair grows from the scalp through a tiny opening called a *follicular orifice*.

The unexposed length of hair underneath the skin's surface is called the *root*. At the end of the root is the hair *bulb* and it is here where cells divide and growth takes place. The *papilla* below the hair bulb is the link between the body's blood supply or source of nourishment, and the hair.

Once hair grows from the scalp, the exposed part is called the *shaft*. If you examine hair underneath a microscope, the outer layer of the hair shaft, the *cuticle*, has microscopic cells called *imbrications* that look like the scales on the trunk of a palm tree. These cuticular cells are clear, though, and their function is to seal in moisture. When hair is damaged (split ends, for example), the cuticle edges become torn and ragged. That's why the texture of dry, damaged hair is rough and brittle.

Under the cuticle is the *cortex*. This is a fibrous structure containing the *pigment* or *melanin*, which gives hair its color. The cortex also contains the protein *keratin*, which is rich in sulfur. Keratin reacts to alkalies like sodium hydroxide, an important chemical used to permanently relax hair. When the

CUTICLE

IMBRICATIONS

HAIR SHAFT

HORNY LAYER

FOLLICLE

SEBACEOUS GLAND

DERMIS

DUCT OF SWEAT GLAND

SWEAT GLAND

ROOT OF HAIR

ARTERY

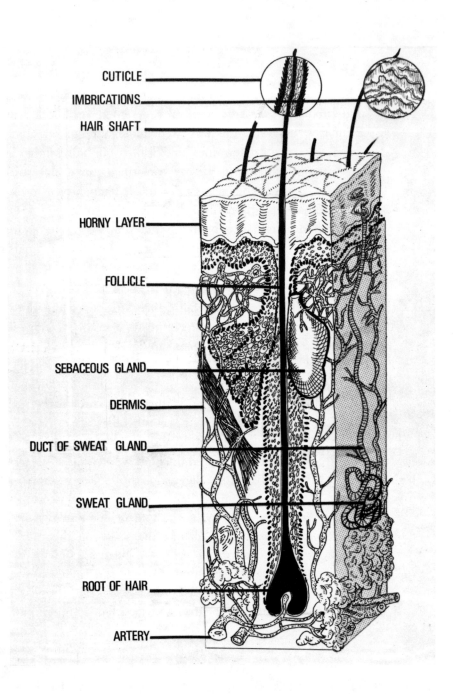

keratin structure is changed, the bonds are rearranged so that curly hair becomes straight.

In the cortex, there are also tiny, individual fibers that are spun into a cable. This weaving gives hair its overall strength and elasticity. Without elasticity, your hair would not stretch, and you could not comb, brush or curl your hair without breaking it.

However, the length that each person's hair stretches varies and this is called the *tensile strength*. When hair is stretched beyond its tensile strength, as often occurs when hair is overrelaxed or set too tightly, it will break. Hair that has been treated with any type of chemical is already stretched and it will snap more easily than hair worn naturally. That's why proper handling at home is so important.

The *medulla* is below the cortex and is the center of the hair shaft. You will only find a medulla in strong hair, never in the hairs around the edges of your scalp. These hairs are called *lanugo,* or soft, fine hairs.

In gray hair, the medulla disappears totally and instead there are tiny bubbles which explains why gray hair is so porous and absorbent. These air bubbles also contribute to the color of gray hair.

WHY IS OUR HAIR FRAGILE? Why is our hair so fragile? Close, tight curls are a natural genetic adaptation to our ancestors' environment. Our alternate curly-wave pattern offers the most effective protection against the sun's penetrating, damaging rays.

If you are wearing your hair in a natural, you can easily see why your hair is so delicate. Pull out one strand and place it on a sheet of white paper. You can see that your curly hair is thick in some places and thinner in others and that it twists wherever it turns to curl. The hair strand is the most fragile where it's thinner or turns to curl.

Often, the tight curls loop into each other and hair tangles easily, so combing must be done gently and correctly (see page 60, "Keeping It Natural").

Not all of our hair has the same curly-wave pattern. Sometimes the curl is close to the scalp, and the ends are wavy. Or, the curl can be at the distal end with waves nearest the scalp. Some of our hair is all wavy, while some has large curls and no waves at all. The combinations and variations of curls and waves are what makes Black hair so unique—and complex.

In curly hair, the root itself is actually curled, too. (This often presents a shaving problem for Black men because it is not easy to catch the hairs near the surface where they begin to curl tightly into the skin.) Straight hair, on the other hand, has a straight root that enters the skin on an angle.

YOUR HAIR'S CYCLE Like everything else in life, hair goes through a cycle. It begins by growing for about four years and this is called the *anagen* stage. The second, transitional stage is called the *catagen* which lasts approximately one week. Afterward it becomes a resting or *telogen* hair and lasts for nearly three months. Once the full cycle is complete, hair falls out.

About 10 to 15 per cent of the hairs on your scalp are in the telogen stage, and dermatologists say you can expect to lose between thirty to sixty of these hairs every day. Washing, combing, or brushing will cause them to separate from the root and fall out. You can easily recognize these hairs because they are club-shaped at the scalp end.

There may be some days when you'll lose very few hairs and other days when you'll lose more. If your hair is long, it may appear as though you are losing an excessive amount, but it's actually the length that makes it seem like a lot. When in doubt, pick up your hairs and count them.

YOUR HEALTH AND YOUR HAIR Excessive hair loss of 150 hairs or more a day may indicate a systemic or internal disorder. Endocrine problems such as thyroid imbalances or diabetes and serious illnesses like cancer or syphilis can cause hair loss even of the eyebrows and eyelashes. Your scalp can warn you of an internal problem, and you should not ignore the signals.

In most cases, however, hair loss is caused by less serious problems. In women, two of the most common are anemia from iron deficiency and that all-too-frequent crash diet. (Hair loss in men is often hereditary and is called *male pattern baldness*.) Also, having a baby, operation, or high fever or beginning or discontinuing any medication including the pill can cause temporary hair loss.

Why? Because the growing hairs are "rushed" into the resting stage due to the hormonal changes occurring in your body, and instead of growing for four years, they complete their entire cycle in the shortened span of a few months. Since it takes a while for you to see the effects of these hormonal changes in your hair, you probably won't notice loss until three or four months following the "trauma."

Such hair loss is only temporary, though, and once your body adjusts your hair loss will decrease. Unless excessive loss persists, don't worry about it.

STRESS   The number-one killer is also the number-one cause of hair loss. Anxiety caused by either environmental or psychological factors can adversely affect your hair.

And, of course, once you begin to worry about your hair loss in addition to agonizing over your problem, you are adding stress on top of stress which only accelerates the hair loss. The immediate remedy is to first solve your problem. Once the stress is alleviated, hair growth will gradually return to normal.

WHAT TO DO   If you suspect that your hair loss is due to an emotional or medical problem, the only thing to do is to seek professional help from your family physician or other specialists such as psychiatrists or dermatologists. Once you make the effort to solve your problem, you will worry less about your hair loss and it will decrease because you recognize that you are on the right road to getting the help you need.

THE SHORT-HAIR SYNDROME   According to Dr. C. Carnot Evans, Jr., Assistant Clinical Professor of Dermatology at Howard University College of Medicine, there are some women whose hair simply will not grow. This is called *pilo tarda* or *Short-hair Syndrome.*

Usually, these women do not have any chemicals in their hair, and they appear to be healthy. Nevertheless, their hair grows to a very short length, then breaks off for no apparent reason.

Mothers who have Short-hair Syndrome often find it in their daughters, too. For this reason, doctors believe that nutrition may be a contributing factor, because mothers who don't eat right don't feed their children correctly, either.

One remedy for SHS, besides having a complete nutritional checkup, is to make certain that anything that comes in contact with the hair is soft and smooth. Pillowcases are a good example. Cotton is extremely abrasive, and satin or nylon pillow cases are much gentler on the hair.

HOT-COMB ALOPECIA   Because we have updated our techniques (see page 64), dermatologists do not see as much Hot-comb Alopecia—baldness resulting from hot oils that melt and burn the scalp—as they did years ago. Nevertheless, this deserves mentioning because if such a burn does occur, the results can be severe. The root structure itself becomes damaged and hair loss is, unfortunately, permanent.

SCALP PROBLEMS   Any bumps, lesions, sores, or hard scales should be checked by a dermatologist immediately. Hair cannot look healthy if there is a problem with the scalp. Again, this may be your first signal of an internal problem.

FREE HAIRCUTS   Hair that breaks off causes nearly as much trauma as hair that falls out. I call these "free haircuts" because we are inadvertently causing the problem ourselves through incorrect handling, hairstyles, and treatments.

UPTURNED COLLARS   You may feel very fashionable when you turn up your jacket, fur- or cloth-coat collar, but before you flip up the collar on your new tweed jacket, realize that our hair is very fragile. The constant contact of any abrasive fabric such as wool or fake fur will pull at your hair in the back and cause it to break.

This is not to say that you should never again wear a high turtleneck sweater, but if your hair is constantly breaking in the center back, or along the ends, you may be wearing high-collar clothing too often.

Also, caps, hats, *galés*, and scarves that are worn too much can break your hair, especially if they are made of cotton, wool, or fake fur. In addition to the fabric catching and pulling your hair out, the tension and pressure of the head covering around the edges of your hairline breaks the fine, lanugo hairs.

If you are in the habit of storing your glasses on top of your head, the pressure of the glasses at your temples may gradually be thinning your hair. Keep your glasses on your nose or in their case.

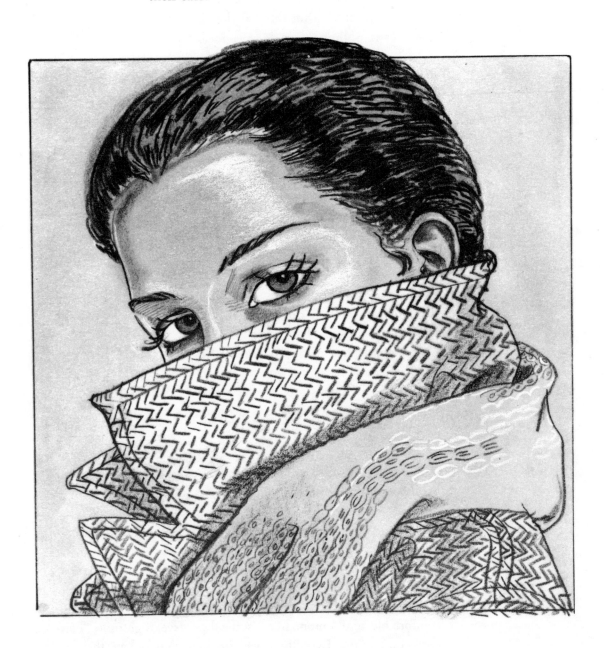

BUNS, BRAIDS, AND BALD SPOTS The hairstyle that is the easiest to manage may not necessarily be the best for your hair. Braiding, plaiting, cornrows, ponytails, and buns that twist and pull your hair too tightly can result in severe hair loss, warns Dr. Evans.

The medical term for this hair loss is *traction alopecia*. Traction means pulling, and alopecia means baldness. Tight hairstyles can pull the hair right out of your scalp—especially at the temples where hair loss takes the shape of a triangle.

Dr. Evans also warns of the dangers of wearing cornrows for too long. Not only does hair loss occur between the cornrows, but there is also total hair loss around the edges of the hairline. Many women who wear cornrows for months and months often have no lanugo hairs at all.

BRUSHING Too much brushing adds to hair loss, especially at the hairline. Even if hair is relaxed, the lanugo hairs grow in curly, and they can be pulled out by harsh brushing. Since hair is often brushed a lot to make a tight, sleek bun in the back, there's double trouble. If you prefer sleek hairstyles, make sure there is enough slack so you can easily move all your hair along the hairline. And avoid a lot of brushing.

If alopecia has not been present for a long time, hair can, and will, grow back, but you must stop doing anything to your hair that puts any stress on the roots. Don't braid or pull it tightly. Wear loose hairstyles and the edges will gradually grow back in.

ROLLERS THAT SPONGE OFF YOUR HAIR More prevalent is hair breakage because of sponge rollers. They actually cling to hair. The soft, spongy surface adheres to individual strands like glue and when you take the rollers out you are taking your own hair out as well.

Sponge rollers cause major damage to our hair, and we should *never* use them. Mesh or smooth plastic rollers are best.

Sleeping in rollers—*any kind of rollers*—besides being uncomfortable and unromantic, is the best free nighttime "haircut" you can get. Every time you turn on your pillow, the friction between the pillow, the roller, and your hair causes the strands of hair to snap.

Keeping your style between shampoos, without ever sleeping in rollers, is probably the biggest challenge of all. But there are several quick, easy alternatives. Here is a wonderful solution from my personal hairstylist, Bruce Clark, who has many of New York's top models as his clients at the Louis M Salon.

A NIGHTTIME PIN-CURL SET
The tightness of your style depends on how many pin curls you make. If you want a loose set, use larger sections of hair. Pin curls should be set in the direction you want your hair to go.

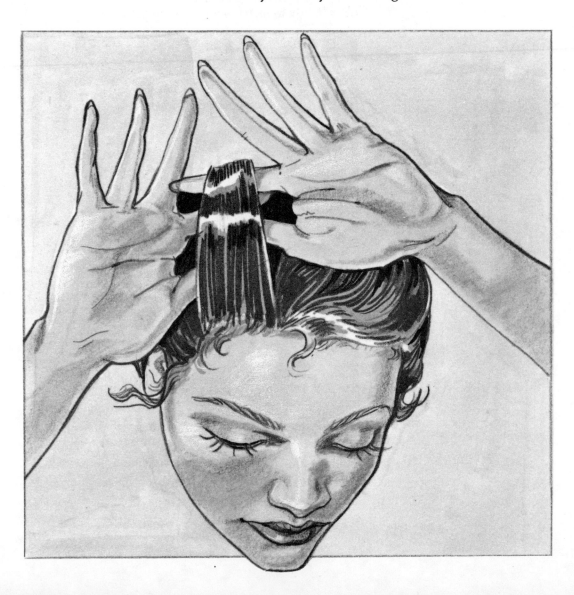

Comb through a section of hair. It is not necessary to part down to the scalp. Wind the hair around your finger and place it against your scalp, laying the curl almost flat. Using a bobby pin (do not sleep in metal clips), secure the end of the curl. Don't pin the stem or you'll flatten your curl. The bobby pin should go through the curl, not over it. If you are making large pin curls, you can crisscross two bobby pins to hold the curl firmer.

Cover your hair comfortably, but not too tightly, with a soft hairnet or silk scarf. (Open-weave-mesh hairnets can be purchased at drugstores and beauty-supply outlets. Keep a "wardrobe" of pretty colors handy to match your sleeping gowns.)

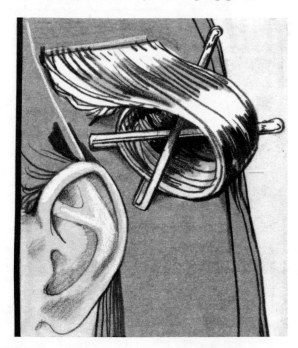

THE SHOWER SET   This pin-curl set also works marvelously in the morning. Just follow all the directions above and cover your hair with a shower cap. The heat from the shower gives you an instant set.

Be sure to allow your hair and body to cool down before taking out the pin curls. It's the combination of the steam and your body heat that gives you such a fast set.

THE MORNING ROLLER SET   Electric rollers are, of course, a quick way for a morning set. Use end papers, though, because the prongs can easily get tangled in your hair. It's not recommended that you use electric rollers too frequently because the constant heat can dry your hair.

In fact, limit use of appliances like blow-dryers and curling wands. These wonderful little gadgets do cut down on otherwise time-consuming tasks, but unless used wisely, they can eventually exact a toll on your hair's luster and condition. If your hair is défrisaged or treated with any chemicals such as a relaxer, overuse of heated appliances can be disaster for you.

Here is Bruce's suggestion for a quick morning set:

QUICK CURLS

Immerse your smooth plastic rollers in very hot water. Let them "set" for five minutes. Remove one at a time and quickly shake off excess water. Set your hair as usual. Put on a shower cap and bathe or shower. Again, the steam sets your hair along with your body heat. Wait a few minutes before removing the rollers.

Stimulate Your Scalp

———•——•——•——•——•——•——•——•——•——•——•——•——•———

What makes hair shiny? Why does our hair look and feel dry? Is oiling the scalp necessary and beneficial? Does it make the hair grow?

The answers in this chapter may surprise you.

WHERE'S THE SHINE? Shine in hair comes from light that is reflected on a flat, smooth surface. Light hits your hair and bounces back to reflect color and shine. In other words, reflected light *is* shine.

Straight hair is flat. Imagine that this hair resembles a long, flat noodle. Light is reflected totally and evenly along the entire length, and hair appears to be very shiny.

Now, take that same imaginary noodle and turn it to make twists and curls like those in curly hair. Wherever there is a turn, the light is interrupted, or refracted, and sent in many different directions. Therefore curly hair appears to look dry because light is not reflected evenly.

Occasionally, too much moisture escapes from the cuticles wherever hair turns or twists to curl. This moisture loss makes our hair not only look dry, but feel dry, too.

In addition, the scalp's natural oils cannot reach the ends of our hair because of the many tight curls. These oils are held on the scalp and cannot distribute themselves to the very ends of the hair. This is another reason why our hair is dry, especially if hair is worn naturally. When hair is thermal pressed or relaxed, the natural oils can reach the ends of the hair more easily.

Oils that are thin and lightweight in texture can help with sealing moisture in very dry hair. Use a small amount, no more than the size of a pea; massage it between the palms of your hands and smooth lightly through your hair.

DISPELLING THE MYTH   Because our hair is dry, we believe that our scalps, too, are dry. Yet, many Black women have normal to oily skin, and it is impossible to have both an oily face and a dry scalp.

Putting oil, pomades, or any substance containing petrolatum or waxes onto the scalp to eliminate this "dryness" is a tradition dating back to the days when our grandmothers and great-grandmothers wanted to maintain a thermal press, says Barbara Ruffin of Black Hair Is, in New York City. But according to dermatologists, this is one of the worst things we can do to both our hair and scalp. Chemicals and perfumes in these oils combine with our own natural oils and can cause scalp irritation.

POMADE ACNE   Not only is the scalp infected, but the forehead also breaks out in blackheads and whiteheads. These pimples can even spread along the sides of the face, and dermatologists call this *Pomade Acne*. The oils that are put onto the hair and scalp are actually causing irritation. When the oils are discontinued, the irritation and acne often clear up.

NOT FOR DANDRUFF EITHER   Oil on the scalp does not control dandruff. This is just another myth. In fact, pomades and oils actually contribute to the dandruff problem.

In most cases, dandruff is the result of a very oily scalp and is called *Seborrheic Dermatitis*. The answer to dandruff is not more oils, but more frequent shampooing. A medicated shampoo that contains sulfur, salicylic acid, protein, and conditioners will control flaking and itching yet leave hair manageable.

The skin and scalp normally shed dead skin cells, and this process is called *exfoliation*. With dandruff, these cells clump together and form large flakes, and because there is the additional factor of hair which traps them, we notice it more than on any other part of our bodies. Adding oil to these already large flakes compounds the problem. When the oil dries on the scalp, it mixes and adheres to the exfoliated cells, causing even larger flakes.

Additionally, the pores get clogged and the scalp just can't breathe, so itching results. The more oil applied, the more itching, dandruff, and irritation there will be.

STIFLING HAIR GROWTH   Pomades and oils on the scalp stifle hair growth. The reproductive process beneath the scalp ·is interfered with because the hair follicle itself is choked by the oils and cannot reproduce normally. Hair growth is slow and minimal. Hair grows twice as fast on a scalp that is never oiled.

OIL YOUR SCALP—NATURALLY   Never oil your scalp artificially—even if it is dry. Frequent shampooing helps wash away the exfoliated cells and deep-conditioning treatments help lubricate the scalp.

Best of all, you have at your fingertips the most natural, totally effective way to encourage your scalp to produce its own oils. *Massage* is the answer. It is great for the body and equally beneficial to your scalp.

HOW DOES MASSAGE WORK?   *Sebaceous* glands are present all over the body, especially the upper arms, chest, back, face, and scalp. The purpose of these glands is to provide the skin and scalp with oil, which is called *sebum*. Massage increases your circulation by bringing more blood to the scalp, which stimulates your sebaceous glands to produce more sebum.

New York hair-care specialist Ron Lee, son of the proprietor of Don Lee Studios, explains how to scalp massage correctly. This is a wonderful favor to exchange with someone you love!

HOW TO MASSAGE YOUR SCALP

Using the fleshy part of your fingertips, place them at the temple area on both the left and right sides of the scalp. Begin the massage by pushing the entire scalp upward, toward the center of the cranium. Make sure the scalp is moved over the cranium and not the hair against the scalp. This can cause breakage. Move the hair and the scalp together, upward, hold for a few seconds, then release. Repeat several times. You will feel the blood flow right down the center of your scalp.

After you've pushed the sides of the scalp toward the top of the cranium, place the palm of one hand on the forehead and the other at the base of the neck. Now, push up again, toward the center of the cranium. Hold for a few seconds, then release. Repeat several times.

Next, working in sections (the back, sides, middle, and top), take the fleshy part of your fingertips and grasp an area of the scalp firmly. Move the scalp over the cranium in small, circular motions. As you're massaging, apply pressure, release, then apply pressure again.

Extend the massage to the surrounding areas, like the forehead and upper and middle back. This will loosen up all the tension that may be causing the glands and muscles to constrict. When the massage is complete, your entire scalp will tingle!

To redistribute these oils to the very ends of your hair, take a rubber-bristled brush (the smooth, rounded bristles will not scratch your scalp or break your hair) and gently brush from the scalp to the ends. Hair will have a natural luster. Brushing also stimulates scalp circulation in addition to removing dead cells, dust, and dirt. Excessive brushing, though, like one hundred strokes, can damage and break fine, delicate hair.

Massage your scalp about once a week. You will be surprised at the amount of oil the body has in reserve. Your hair will look healthier and shinier in a short period of time.

PRECAUTIONS If you have blood-pressure problems, heart or other circulatory problems, do not massage your scalp. You do not want to increase the circulation of blood to your head.

Also, if you have any cuts or pimples on the scalp itself, do not massage. First, see a dermatologist.

SMOKE GETS IN YOUR HAIR Smoke not only restricts the circulation of your entire body, it also restricts the circulation of blood to your scalp. If you can't quit smoking for your heart's sake, do it for your hair's.

Something New About Shampoo

Cosmetically, hair looks best when just shampooed. It is its shiniest, bounciest, freshest. And when your hair looks good, you feel good, so you want to maintain your hair in its optimum condition as often as possible.

HOW OFTEN SHOULD YOU SHAMPOO? If you live in metropolitan areas where hair is subjected to more pollutants than in suburban areas, you'll want to shampoo at least every four or five days; seven days is the absolute maximum. Sebum, combined with the pollutants in our environment, may produce odor after more than a few days. Also, frequent shampooing washes away exfoliated cells, which prevents itching and flaking.

If you feel you need to shampoo every three days or every two days, then do so. Daily shampooing is still impractical and often unnecessary. In fact, dermatologists and hairstylists consider it harmful. Your hair and scalp need the sebaceous oils, so why wash them away every day? If you have an oily scalp, this condition is only aggravated by too frequent shampooing, because the process of shampooing itself actually stimulates the oil glands. The result—an even oilier scalp.

GETTING THE CHLORINE OUT There are exceptions, of course—occasions when you may want to shampoo daily. If you are on vacation and are swimming every day, the salt water and chlorine are extremely drying to your hair. It is absolutely necessary to shampoo immediately after swimming. If you enjoy water sports, be sure to condition your hair frequently, too.

CHOOSING YOUR SHAMPOO Since it's impractical to visit a salon every time you're ready for a shampoo, home hair care and choosing the right products are very important.

Select a shampoo designed for treated hair if your hair is relaxed or thermal-pressed, or a shampoo for delicate hair if yours is natural. In addition, your shampoo should be geared to your individual hair type—dry, normal, or oily.

If your hair feels rough or brittle soon after you shampoo, then it is dry. Oily hair has an oily film a day or two following shampoo, while normal hair is easy to manage between shampoos.

Your shampoo should be pH balanced so that your hair will be smooth, easy to comb, and manageable. The symbol pH refers to the level of alkaline and acid, and the scale is from 0 to 14, with 0 being highly acidic and 14 highly alkaline. If hair becomes too alkaline, it will be too porous. The cuticle scales of the hair "open," and hair becomes frizzy, coarse, and unruly. However, shampoos that have a balanced pH level neutralize the alkaline and "close" the cuticles on the hair shaft. Before you buy, check labels for a pH range of 4.5 to 5.5.

In addition to a balanced pH level, shampoo should contain *hydrolyzed animal proteins.* This is extremely important and guarantees you the best quality shampoo for your hair. Hydrolyzed protein is water soluble; each molecule is so tiny that it can actually be absorbed into the hair shaft.

ALL SHAMPOOS ARE NOT ALIKE How can you tell if a shampoo is right for you? The texture and feel of your hair both when it is wet and when it is dry are your best indicators. Be very objective. Does your hair feel very mushy when it's wet? You probably have a shampoo that is leaving a heavy coating on your hair. Does it feel brittle and coarse? The shampoo may contain too many detergents for you.

If you travel frequently, remember that water changes ("soft" and "hard") from region to region, and this may affect the performance of your shampoo.

Ask your stylist to recommend products for you. Perhaps you might like to continue your salon regimen at home and use products that are complementary to your salon treatments. Finding the right shampoo is imperative for beautiful-looking hair.

SUDSING UP Hairstylist Bruce Clark recommends using two shampoos. First, one to clean your hair and scalp. You can easily tell if this shampoo is really cleaning; your scalp will tingle, feel really alive, and hair will feel crisp and clean. The caution here: Don't overdo it. Usually one lather is plenty. Besides the excellent commercial brands available, you may want to check health-food stores for natural, peppermint-type *cleansing shampoos* to see which works best for you.

The second lather should be with a *conditioning shampoo*. It combines the softening agents of a cream rinse which detangles hair. And it can have built-in conditioners like balsams or proteins, plus the cleansing properties of a shampoo. Conditioning shampoos can be used with or without cleansing shampoos, but they do not take the place of a deep-conditioning treatment.

Demand a lot from this second shampoo. It should make your hair *look* good, with a natural shine that lasts until your next shampoo. Hair should be manageable and easy to comb after just one lather of your conditioning shampoo.

Here are Bruce's instructions for the correct way to shampoo your hair.

HOW TO SHAMPOO HAIR THAT IS SHOULDER-LENGTH OR SHORTER

Measure about one capful of *cleansing* shampoo into the palms of your hands. Work the shampoo into a soft lather and gently smooth it onto your wet hair. Once it's applied, take the fleshy part of your fingertips and firmly massage the scalp, using tiny, circular motions, working all hair in the same direction. Do the top of the scalp, crown area, base of the scalp, and sides. Rinse thoroughly. Lather again with same amount of *conditioning shampoo*. Rinse thoroughly and comb through gently with a wide-tooth comb. The final rinse should be with cool water, which helps close the cuticle so hair is smooth and shiny.

HOW TO SHAMPOO LONG HAIR

Follow the same directions as above. Apply the shampoo only to the scalp, not to the ends of your hair. The shampoo will naturally distribute itself to the ends. Never take your hair and pull it to the top of your head to scrub it against the rest of your hair. This will cause breakage. Also, rubbing the hair harshly between the palms of your hands will cause it to tangle. Hair at the ends is oldest and more fragile, so just smooth excess suds along the hair in one direction to gently clean it.

SHAMPOO RULES:

Always . . .

Lather twice, depending on how oily your hair is. It isn't necessary to shampoo until hair is "squeaky clean." If hair squeaks, it is usually overshampooed and can look dry and brittle as a result.

Rinse out shampoo thoroughly. A good rule is to rinse three times as long as you shampoo.

Finish your rinsing with cool water. This helps close the imbrications on the hair shaft so that hair reflects light better. It will be softer and look shinier.

Comb through wet hair with a wide-tooth comb only. Small teeth will not glide through hair easily. They will cause hair to snap wherever there are tangles.

Clean combs and brushes as often as you shampoo.

Never . . .

Take the bottle and squeeze the shampoo directly onto your hair. Too much shampoo may leave a soapy residue and hair can look dry and dull.

Scrub your scalp with your nails or with any kind of brush. You can scratch and irritate your scalp.

Force the comb through your hair. If it offers any kind of resistance, you need to use a cream rinse following your conditioning shampoo. Be sure to rinse out thoroughly.

Brush wet hair. All hair is very fragile when wet, and the slightest tension will cause it to snap.

HOW TO COMB WET HAIR   Wet hair is fragile. Water changes the molecular arrangement of keratin and each individual strand of hair can stretch very easily. If you put too much tension on it when drying or combing, the strands can easily snap.

When you emerge dripping from shower or sink, never but never take a towel and rub your hair vigorously! The towel can actually tear your hair. Instead, wrap your head for a few minutes and let the towel absorb the moisture.

Comb though your hair completely with a wide-tooth comb or with your metal pick if you are wearing a natural. Remember never to force the comb through your hair. Your conditioning shampoo should leave your hair virtually tangle-free. If it hasn't, use a cream rinse. If you use a spray-type cream rinse, it is not necessary to rinse it out.

To comb wet hair, gently ease out any remaining tangles by slowly beginning with the hair that's closest to your scalp. Comb through to the ends, section by section. If your hair is very tangled, gently comb the ends first and work up toward the scalp.

Once you've combed through completely you are ready to condition or set and style your hair.

The Condition You're In

Conditioning your hair is important for maintaining body, luster, and manageability. To keep your hair looking its best, you should supplement your regular salon visits with deep-conditioning treatments at home.

WHY A CONDITIONER? Normal combing, brushing, and general handling can damage the imbrications on the outer layer of the hair shaft. If they become become torn or rough, they can snag against each other, causing your hair to break. Conditioners help smooth the hair shaft by closing the cuticle and, in some cases, temporarily mend split ends by filling in the spaces. Conditioners minimize friction and static electricity when you comb your hair, and leave hair smooth, soft, and shiny.

TWICE A MONTH IS ENOUGH If your hair is in good, healthy condition, twice a month is enough for a deep-conditioning at-home treatment. If your hair is damaged, you should give yourself a treatment once every week for about two months or until your hair is back to normal, then switch to every other week.

If you have a relaxer, thermal press your hair, or have any color treatments in it, you may want to condition your hair more frequently than twice a month. Once hair is removed from its natural state, it requires a little more pampering and attention to guard against damage. Once-a-week treatments are best.

TRAVEL AND TREATMENTS Being constantly on the go means that your conditioner should be one that requires as few ingredients and as little mixing as possible. When you shop for that conditioner, try to find one that's geared to your type of hair. Use the same criteria as you do in selecting your shampoo.

Conditioning your hair while you're on the beach is a wonderful way to maximize the heat of the sun while protecting your hair from it's damaging rays. Once you finish sunning, remember to rinse the conditioner completely out of your hair. Instant conditioners that are sprinkled onto the scalp and left there, for instance, may cause the scalp to flake once it has dried. If you do use an instant conditioner, be sure to put it only on your hair.

AT-HOME TREATMENTS   Here are a few at-home deep-conditioning treatments from top salons. Next to each of the conditioning treatments listed are recommendations for the type of hair for which they are best suited. For example, if you have split ends, deep conditioners for damaged hair are what you need to help seal the ends together. Oil conditioners help restore oil to both dry hair and scalp.

Observe how your hair looks and feels between treatments, then decide if you want to continue the regimen. You should notice the difference in your hair after your very first treatment, but since the effects of any conditioner are temporary, you will have to repeat the treatment as often as you feel necessary.

Following the list of treatments are Bruce's instructions for applying your conditioner.

CONDITIONING TREATMENTS FROM TOP NEW YORK SALONS

1. *THE LOUIS M SALON.* Recommended for all hair, to add luster and manageability, by Bruce Clark.

You will need:

One 1.9 ounce tube of Wella Kolestral Concentrate Molasses

Mix:

The entire tube of Kolestral with an equal amount of molasses until the color is a medium brown. The molasses helps the Kolestral penetrate the hair shaft. This is a good weekly treatment.

2. *EL YUNQUE OBA.* Recommended, to add shine and body to dry hair, by Ruth Sanchez Laviera.

You will need:

Oleocap by L'Oréal, Deep Penetrating Precious Oil Treatment For Dry Hair–five-application box. Follow directions on box.

Note:

After heating oil, make sure it isn't too hot by testing on the inside of your wrist before applying to your hair.

3. *ANTOINE FELIPE SALON*. Recommended, for very dry hair and scalp, by Conrad Symister.

You will need:

1 raw egg
½ cup mayonnaise
½ teaspoon olive oil

Mix well.

Note:

This treatment should be applied to clean hair but you will have to shampoo again—two or three additional lathers–to shampoo the treatment out completely.

4. *HAIRSTYLING BY JOSEPH*. Recommended, for dry, brittle, or damaged hair, by Joseph Plaskett.

You will need:

Olive oil
Coconut oil
Odorless castor oil
Vitamin E liquid

Mix:

Equal parts, enough for one treatment.

Note:

Apply *before* shampoo. You will need at least two or three lathers to remove all of the oil.

PREPARATION FOR YOUR CONDITIONING TREATMENT

You will need:

Cleansing and conditioning shampoos.

A medium-size towel, cut in half, lengthwise, measuring about forty inches long and ten inches wide. It will allow you enough towel to completely cover your hair yet it is small enough to fit under your heat cap or dryer.

A plastic shower cap.

A heat cap. The plastic hooded caps insulated with wire to generate heat are used in most salons and are a valuable beauty investment. You can purchase one at any beauty-supply outlet. Or, you can substitute one at home by using a plastic shower cap and sitting under a hooded dryer.

Timer

Conditioning treatment

Wide-tooth comb

Now you are ready to:

1. Soak your towel in very hot tap water.

2. Shampoo hair with cleansing and conditioning shampoos. Blot excess water.

3. Evenly distribute the conditioner to the outer edges of your hair first—around the temples, front, sides, and nape—because this is where the fine, lanugo hairs are. They are the most delicate and take the most abuse from brushing and combing, so need conditioning the most.

4. Starting at the back, apply the conditioner to your scalp, then to the entire hank or section of hair. Continue to sides and top.

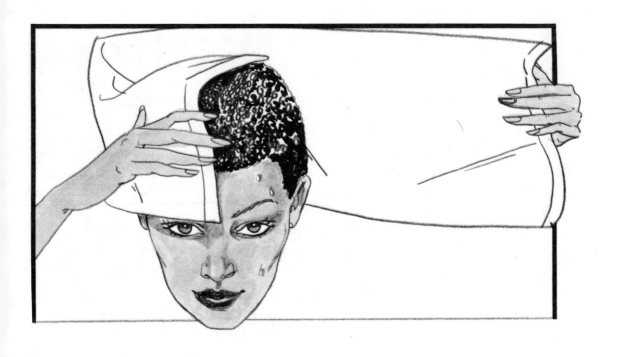

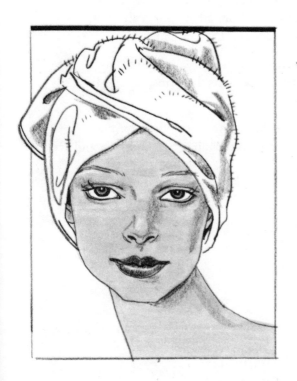

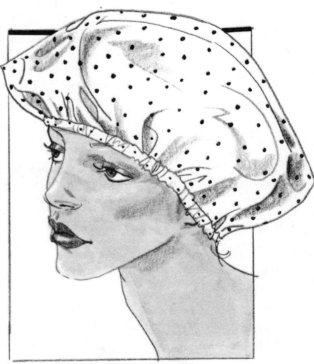

5. Once all of the conditioner is applied, gently massage it into your scalp, using the fleshy part of your fingertips.

6. Comb through gently with a wide-tooth comb.

7. Remove the towel from the hot water and wring it until it is just damp. Wrap your head so that all your hair is covered. Secure by tucking the ends in. Do not us any pins because this can be dangerous when heat is applied.

8. Put on your plastic shower cap. Sit under your dryer or heat cap, and set the timer for twenty-five minutes.

9. When treatment is finished, rinse hair thoroughly with very warm water. Do not comb through your hair until most of the conditioner has been rinsed out because hair is very soft and breakable at this point.

10. Rinse again, massaging the scalp to make sure the conditioner is removed from all of your scalp area, including the temples and back of hair.

11. Rinse a third time, this time combing through with a wide-tooth comb. This final rinse should be with cool water.

12. Dry or set hair following instructions for natural, thermal-pressed, or relaxed hair. (See "Styling and Treatments.")

Coloring Adds Warmth and Richness

· ·

For Black women, luminous hair color adds richness to an already beautiful skin tone. And coloring the hair, which can make any woman look younger and more attractive, is not just limited to women who want to cover the gray. Giving your hair a warm, soft shade is a wonderful way to gently highlight your hair, your face, your eyes.

A WARM SHAMPOO   Shampoo-in hair color is an easy, single-process tint that gives you the best guarantee of an even, predictable color that will last. Internationally acclaimed colorist Leslie Blanchard, proprietor of The Private World of Leslie Blanchard in New York City, says that even for covering gray hair, warm, golden tones of brown are particularly beautiful for our skin. Shades that are too light or too dark can look artificial.

The first time you decide to color your hair, Leslie suggests you choose a shade that is very close to your own natural hair color. Are you thinking about a dramatic change? First, try on a wig in your "new" color to see if it actually does flatter you. Remember, the more dramatic your new hair color, the larger your money and time investments will be to maintain your new look.

AN EXCITING CONDITION   For exciting hair color, always condition your hair regularly, advises Leslie. Remember to condition the ends of your hair, which are the most porous areas, several days before coloring your hair. Conditioning seals the cuticles, preventing the cortex from absorbing too much color.

Shampoo-in hair color should be applied to the roots or new growth first. During the last few minutes, shampoo the ends. If you relax your hair, wait three to four weeks before you color.

DON'T DOUBLE UP   The double-process hair color, or dyeing your hair, can be too harsh on fragile, delicate hair. It often contains strong chemicals (bleach) to first strip the hair of its original color before adding another shade (dye).

The double process sometimes causes systemic problems such as a feeling of general malaise. In more severe cases, reactions can vary from breaking out in pimples and sores to a swollen, balloonlike face.

To avoid such allergic reactions, called *contact dermatitis,* always give yourself a strand patch test before coloring your hair. Apply the color to the side of your hair in the back and wait twenty-four to forty-eight hours. If you have a bad reaction, see your doctor or dermatologist *immediately.*

COLORING HAIR WITH HENNA   For thousands of years, henna has been a popular method of coloring and highlighting hair. Henna is made from the powdered leaves of a tropical plant found mainly in the Middle East.

Some experts say different species of henna plants give us different colors. Others believe each section of the plant has its own, pure color. The root gives us a deep black, the leaves a vibrant red, and from inside the stem comes neutral henna.

Colors and tones vary according to the age of the plant, and shades can be mixed and blended to create dramatic effects. Your hair-color results, though, are often unpredictable. They are also permanent. Always give yourself a strand test before your henna treatment.

ON THE OUTSIDE, SEALING IN   Henna does not penetrate into the cortex layer. It acts as a sealer, coating the hair shaft in an effort to lock in moisture. However, henna should not be used on porous, frizzy, or damaged hair. In its effort to seal in moisture, henna will seal the cuticles open and hair will be coarse and hard to comb.

If your hair has been relaxed, wait two weeks following your treatment before you henna your hair. By then, the cuticles should be closed again.

NOT FOR GRAY HAIR   Henna should never be used on hair that is more than 20 per cent gray. Gray hair is very porous and the henna

will seep into the cuticles and alter the hair's pigment dramatically. The result may be an orangey-red color that is difficult,
often impossible, to correct.

Never henna your hair if you have a shampoo-in color, and
never color your hair over a henna.

CONDITION BEFORE AND AFTER   Conrad Symister of the Antoine
Felipe Salon in New York City recommends conditioning your
hair twice in order to enjoy the full benefits of your henna
treatment.

Condition before, to restore protein and close the cuticles.
Condition afterward, to seal in the effects of your henna treatment.

SAFE AT HOME   Henna is safe to use at home, but mixing and applying
the powder can make application a bit messy. Conrad suggests
the following for your at-home henna treatment.

HOW TO HENNA AT HOME

Before you begin, protect your hands from staining by
wearing rubber gloves. Cover your shoulders with a
smock or old shirt and a towel, too.

Coat the edges of your hairline with a petrolatum
or wax base pomade to protect your face from
staining.

Keep plenty of moistened paper towels handy to
catch drips on face, shoulders, or neck. Newspaper
the floor to protect it from spills.

Shampoo and condition your hair. Without setting
your hair, let it dry under a hooded dryer for
approximately fifteen minutes, depending on the
length and thickness of your hair. Do not blow-dry.

Section your hair in two, parting from the center
front to the center nape. Clip one section out of the
way.

Following package directions, mix henna in a
stainproof or glass bowl using very hot water. (It
should not be boiling because you could burn your
scalp.)

Using a tint brush, while the henna is hot apply it to the loose section, beginning at the center part at the bottom. Working upward, apply henna to the roots of your hair first. Make lengthwise parts and continue to apply until the entire half is completed. Repeat on opposite side.

To bring the paste to the ends of your hair, take the fleshy part of your rubber-gloved fingertips and gently massage, making sure all your hair is covered. If your hair is long, secure the ends together at the top with a hairpin or bobby pin. Henna the remaining section.

Once the entire hair is covered, wrap a paper towel, folded in half, along the nape of your neck, up and around to cover your ears and forehead.

Cover your head securely with a plastic shower cap or bag and sit under a heat cap or warm hooded dryer for about forty-five minutes.

With very warm water, rinse your hair thoroughly. Use your fingertips to help loosen any part of the paste that may have dried on your scalp. Don't forget the edges and back. Rinse again.

Shampoo with your cleansing shampoo to remove all traces of the henna. Follow with your conditioning shampoo.

Condition hair and set, following instructions for natural, thermal-pressed, or relaxed hair. (See "Styling and Treatments.")

Styling and Treatments

The Right Style and Treatment for You

• — • — • — • — • — • — • — • — • — • — • — • — • — • — • — • — • — •

Black hair is the most incredible hair there is! It can be worn naturally or relaxed permanently, temporarily, or just partially. Whatever we decide to do, it's not because of imitations, but because we have no limitations.

This section discusses your styling options with specific instructions on the best home treatments. The basis, of course, is a good haircut, and you will be given guidelines to help you and your stylist choose a cut that's right for you, whether your hair is natural, relaxed, or défrisaged.

Illustrations tell you how to cornrow your hair and how to make individual braids as long as you like. Twisting and rolling your hair are other pretty options you can choose, too.

Tips on the most handy beauty accessory from a talented young designer plus an innovator's peek into the future of our hair are also included.

[*Note:* Hair in the photographs in this section personally styled by each featured hairstylist.]

The Shape Is In the Cut

Next to a hairstylist you can trust, scissors are your hair's best friend. You cannot have a beautiful hairstyle no matter how well you shampoo, condition, and set your hair, unless it is shaped properly. And no matter how you wear your hair—natural, relaxed, or défrisaged—the shape comes from the cut.

Here's where you rely on your hairstylist the most. He or she should take a good look at you while you're standing to get an overall view of you. Now in shaping your hair, your stylist can consider your proportions and give you a cut that complements your bone structure as well as your facial features.

Your hairstylist should also ask you questions about your lifestyle. Do you love spending hours fussing with your hair or is the least bit of effort the most you can handle? Your answers should influence his decision in choosing the perfect style for you.

SPLITTING HAIRS Split ends are inevitable since hair at the ends is the oldest and has been handled—brushed, combed, set, braided—the most. The frizzed, damaged part can extend up the entire hair shaft or get caught in your comb or brush and break. To prevent this, you will need a trim every six to eight weeks to snip them off. Trimming also maintains the shape of your haircut as your hair grows longer.

To determine if you're ready for a trim, comb your wet hair so that it forms a bowl shape around your face with the center at the crown area. Can you still follow the line of your original cut? If not, it's time for a trim.

PATTING IT TOGETHER Naturals may have to be trimmed more often, like every four weeks, because the style is so dependent on a well-defined line. Once you have to pat your Afro into the shape you want, you know you're ready for your stylist to even the ends. If you're adept, you may even be able to give yourself a trim at home. (See "Keeping It Natural" for how-to instructions.)

THE "EYES" HAVE IT Before you and your stylist decide on the haircut that's best for you, pull all your hair back and take a good look at your face. What shape is it? Is your face oval with prominent cheekbones? Or is it round with fleshy cheeks? Is it long or do you have a very broad, defined jawline so that your face is square-shaped?

Of course you want to bring the most attention to your eyes and your cheekbone area, and your hairstyle, along with your makeup, should work together to help create the illusion of big eyes.

Master cutter Eric Turner of the Cinandre Salon in New York City offers these guidelines to help you emphasize your eyes through your haircut and style. These are not rules, just suggestions, since faces can be combinations of shapes such as long and square or long and oval, for instance.

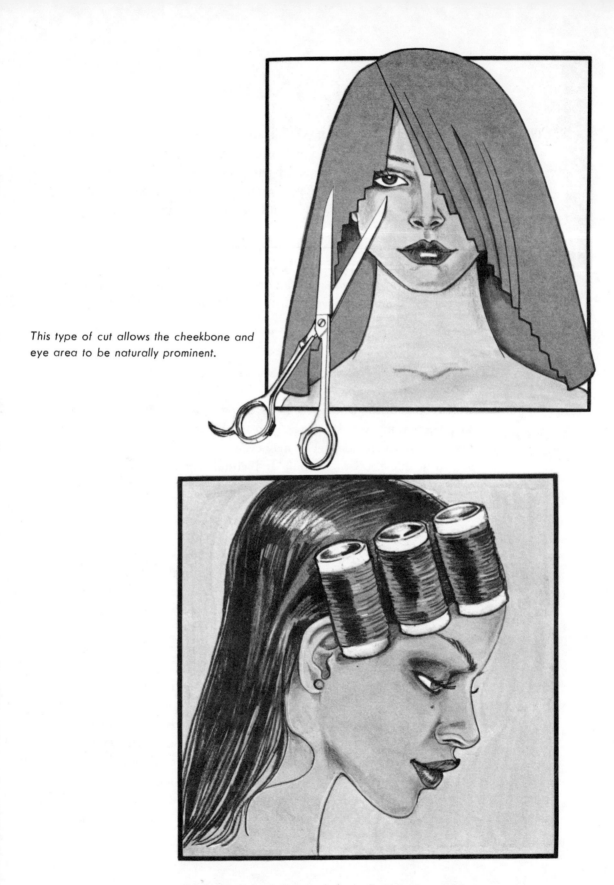

This type of cut allows the cheekbone and eye area to be naturally prominent.

Setting the sides on an angle away from the face add even more dimension to the oval-shaped face. The remainder of the hair is set following the same angle. Here, plastic rollers are used, eliminating the need for end papers.

The comb out—soft, smooth, and off the face for the most dramatic eyes.

Cut, set, and style, Bruce Clark

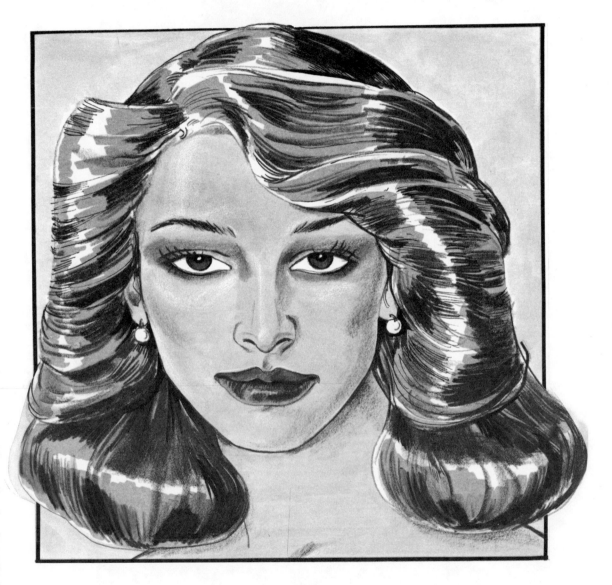

AN OVAL FACE   Emphasis is already in the cheek and eye area, and you want your hair to blend in with your face shape, not distract from it. Styles that frame your face like a bathing cap are most flattering if your hair is short. If it is long, keep your hairstyle soft, sleek, and simple, with hair shortest at the cheek area so that you make the most of what you have.

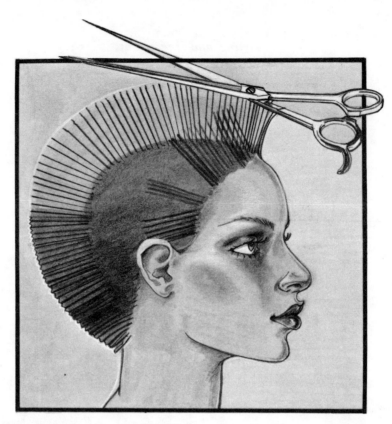

This illustrates how hair should be cut shortest at the nape, longer at the sides and top.

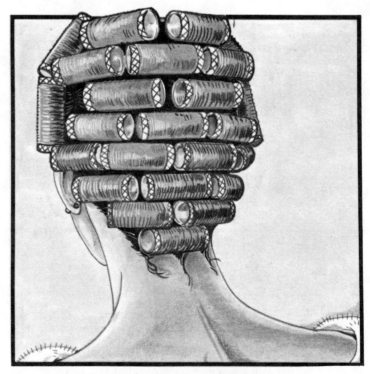

The zigzag set means that you are not going to have long lines of parts to camouflage. Each row naturally blends in with the part below it. Here, mesh rollers and end papers were used.

The comb out—beautifully proportioned, with hair combed off the face to really open it up. The wider sides give the illusion of broad cheekbones; the high crown adds needed length.

Cut, set, and style, Bruce Clark

A ROUND FACE   Since your face is full right down to the jawline, your cheekbones are not as prominent as in the oval face. Your hairstyles, therefore, should not follow the contour of your face like a bathing cap because this will only make it look rounder. Avoid wearing bangs or bringing any hair over your cheeks. Complementary hairstyles are those that are off your face and fuller at the sides and top. To further thin your face, lift hair up and away from your chin so that the nape is tapered shorter than the rest of your hair.

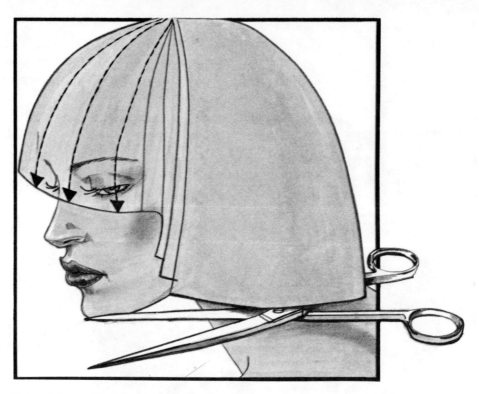

Hair is longer when wet, so this cut for a long face illustrates the general length of bangs. To add width, hair is slightly layered at the sides and bottom.

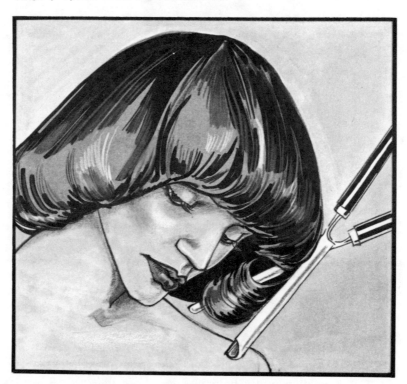

After hair has been thermal-pressed or défrisaged (see "Styling and Treatments"), hair is combed into a bowl shape and the ends are curled under with a curling wand.

The comb out—flattering bangs shorten the long face, and fuller sides create the illusion of prominent cheekbones— and big eyes.

Cut, set, and style, Rose Morgan

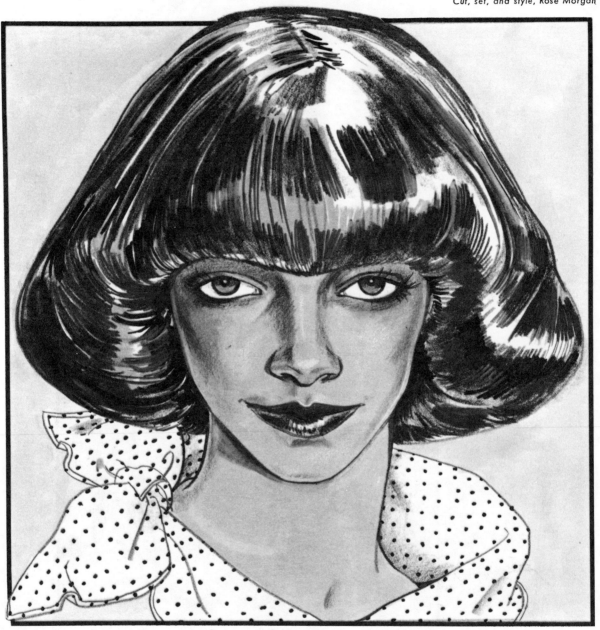

A LONG FACE   There are different areas of your face that may be long, such as your forehead or chin. Your objective is to add balance.

Choose styles with bangs to cut the length of your face. Fullness at the sides gives you the width that's becoming to you. Or fluffy hairstyles that are slightly shorter at the neck and crown but longer at the sides will also create a well-balanced illusion.

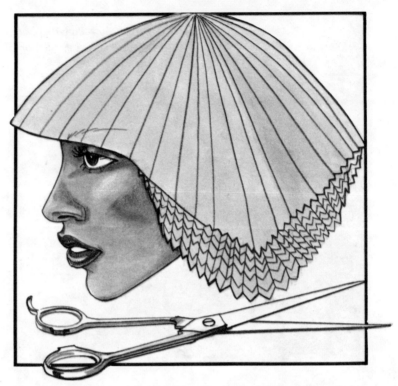

Hair is cut so that it is closely layered to form a triangle with the widest points at the eye and cheekbone area.

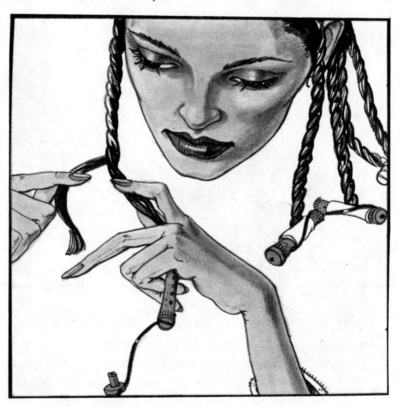

A new set that adds texture to hair is to twist two hanks of hair together, place an end paper at the bottom to prevent ends from frizzing, and roll the ends around a medium-size permanent rod.

The comb out—a crimped style that takes the attention
away from the jawline adds softness to a square face.
This style can be worn two other ways: simply untwist the
locks and let them fall naturally, or comb through with your
fingers or the tail of a rattail comb for looser locks.

Cut, set, and style, Conrad Symister

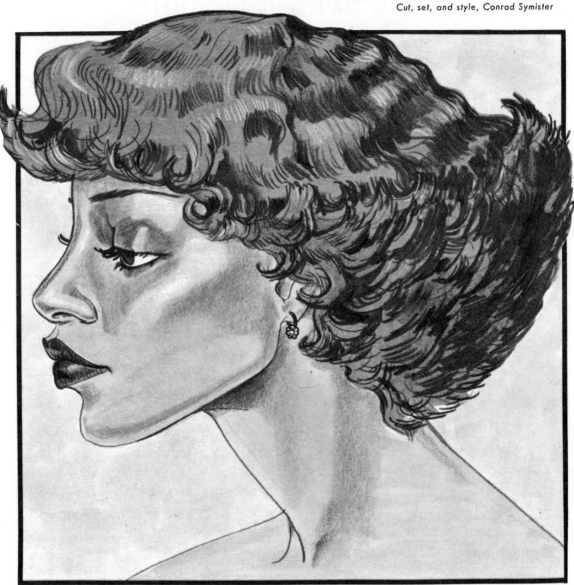

A SQUARE FACE You can't minimize your jaw by covering it up with hair. In fact, this will actually make it more prominent. Hairstyles that allow you to wear straight, fluffed, or side-swept bangs draw the attention upward, giving your face a wonderful balance. Around your chin area, be sure to keep your hair brushed back or off your face altogether.

Keeping It Natural

The birth of the "natural" in America was one of the most revolutionary beauty concepts ever experienced by both Black women and men alike. For the first time, the new awareness of the sixties allowed us to take pride in our hair's natural beauty. Today the aesthetics of texturized hair are evidenced by women of all ethnic groups who proudly sport frizzy permanents and curly body waves.

NEW SINGER IN TOWN Camello Casimir (better known as Frenchie), of the Casdulan Salon in New York City, is renowned as the stylist who first introduced the Afro to America. For a photograph which appeared in the January 1960 issue of *Look* magazine, he distinguished the young African singer, Miriam Makeba, by designing this hairstyle just for her—a style that quickly caught the imagination of Black youth anxious to exemplify their political awareness in the forefront of the Civil Rights Movement.

Popularized as the "Afro" because of Miriam's heritage, Black hair was finally unveiled, defying tradition, stripped of hot combs and chemicals. It was soon interchangeably called the "natural" since it was the first time Black hair was ever styled in its own natural state. So great was the demand that stylists such as Black Rose, famed New York barberist who excelled in cutting, had lines of men and women waiting when she opened her salon doors.

IS IT RIGHT FOR EVERYONE? The natural surprised many by requiring gentler handling than when hair was temporarily or permanently relaxed, and a quick review of "The Right Care for Delicate Hair" explains why.

Are there women who should not wear their hair naturally? Dianne Turner, noted barberist with the Femme Fatale Salon in New York, acknowledges that some textures of hair with very tight curly ends break more easily than textures that have looser curls. The curls get caught in the comb or pick and snap easily. A partially relaxed natural or *Jheri-Curl* is a contemporary natural that minimizes breakage.

WET COMBING   When you comb your natural, and with what, are very important in keeping it beautiful and healthy-looking. The tight curls prevent your scalp's natural oils from reaching the ends and your hair may tend to be dry. To minimize brittleness, always dampen your hair before you comb it, and apply a tiny amount of a lightweight hairdressing to your *wet* hair. Avoid heavy sprays that coat your hair, and again, never oil your scalp.

Gently comb your hair, section by section, then pat so that it is even. Do not try to even your shape all in one stroke. Constantly combing your hair in one direction, from the back to the forehead, for instance, will eventually cause it to thin in the back.

PICKING THE RIGHT PICK   Choosing the right type of hair accessory is vital to your natural, and Dianne offers these suggestions.

Avoid wood or plastic combs or picks because they do not glide through your hair easily. Instead, metal picks with thin prongs, no more than 1/16th of an inch in diameter, comb hair without causing breakage.

Your pick should have at least nine or ten prongs to allow you to comb the entire back of your hair in one motion. If there are fewer prongs, you will break your hair just trying to get it even.

If your hair is long, the prongs in the pick should be at least 4½ inches long. A short pick is fine for short hair, but it will catch long hair and cause it to break.

SHAPING IT UP   To insure a style that complements your features, the initial shaping should be done by a professional. Then, have your natural trimmed every six to eight weeks; four to five weeks if your hair grows quickly. Once you have to pat your hair into shape, you know you're ready for a trim.

If you are steady-handed, you can follow your stylist's shape and trim your own hair at home. Here are Dianne's directions.

HOW TO TRIM YOUR NATURAL

Before you begin to trim your hair, take both hands and feel your head for any protrusions or depressions. Because the actual shape of the head is camouflaged by the thickness of the hair, many women don't realize that one side of their head may be larger than the other.

If there is a protrusion, hair must be longer on the opposite side. Even the protruding side first, then trim the other side to match. If there is a depression in any part of the scalp such as the nape, leave hair in that area slightly longer.

To begin trimming your natural, braid or blow-dry your hair to extend it before cutting.

Use two mirrors—one wall and one hand mirror—so you can easily see the sides and back of your hair.

Use electric clippers *only*. Scissors will give you an uneven line every time you make a new snip.

Begin at the nape, in the center, and trim upward toward the crown in one smooth, steady motion. Repeat for one side, then the other, always working from the back toward the front.

At first, trim just a little, then begin again at the center nape, repeating the entire procedure until your hair is the length you want.

Shampoo and condition your hair. Blot excess water by wrapping hair with a towel. Apply a tiny amount of a lightweight hairdress if necessary. Comb and let dry naturally. Your Afro allows you the luxury of limiting the use of blow-dryers and appliances that can dry your fragile ends. For versatility, braid or twist your hair while it's wet. Let dry, then comb (see page 91).

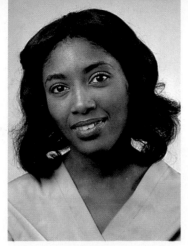

ESTHER DOWNING

Step 1: Before

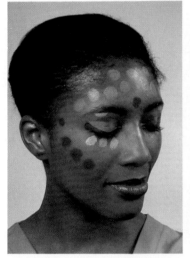

Step 2: Seven steps for makeup

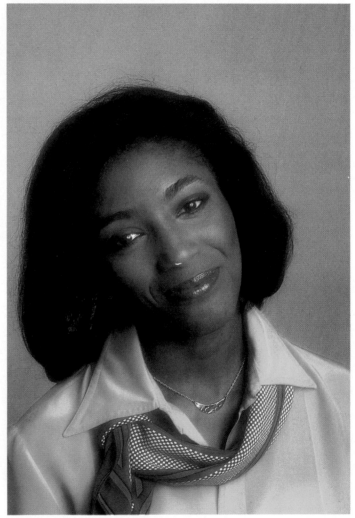

Step 3: Daytime look

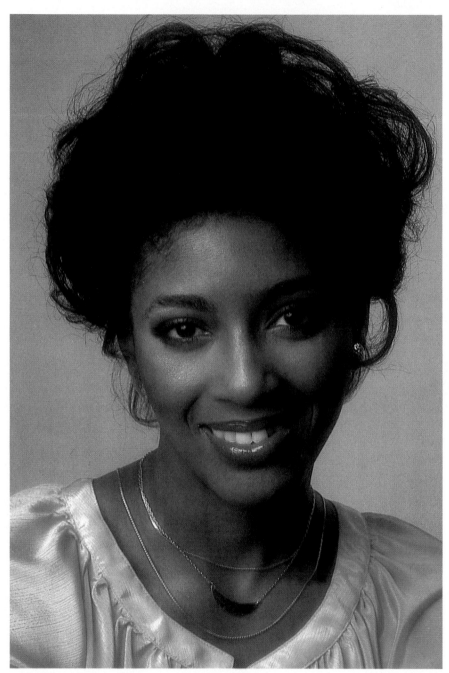

Step 4: Evening drama

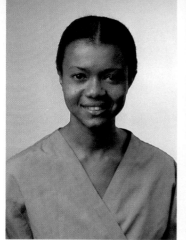

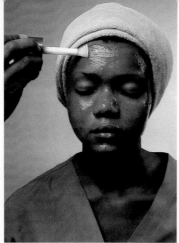

SYLVIA DAVIS

Step 1: Before

Step 2: Applying a facial mask

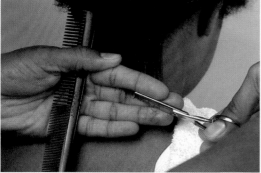

Step 3: Trimming the ends

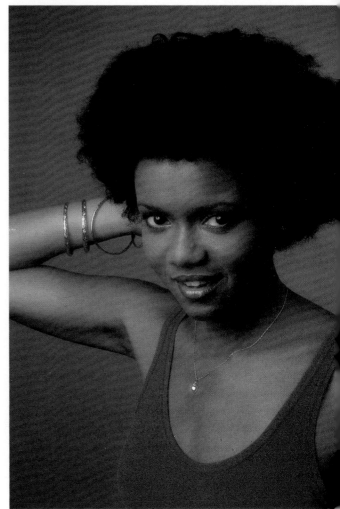

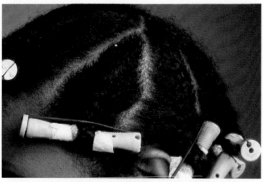

Step 4: Cornrowed and set on perm rods

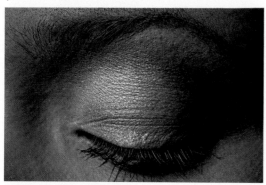

Step 5: Eye makeup

Step 6: After

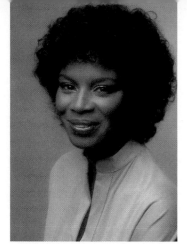

Step 1: Three looks. First,
a sporty wig . . .

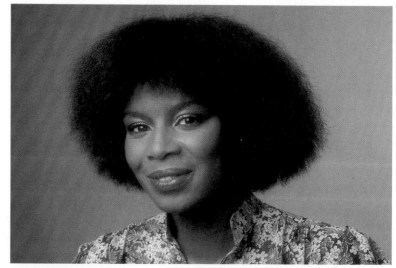

Step 2: Changed to a party look . . .

ARLENE FRIDIE

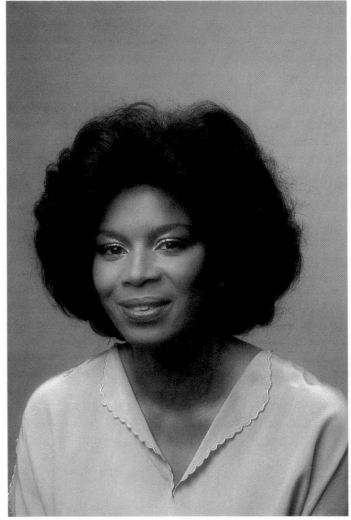

Step 3: Then more sophisticated.

MADELINE CLEARE

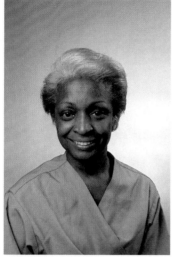

Step 1: Before

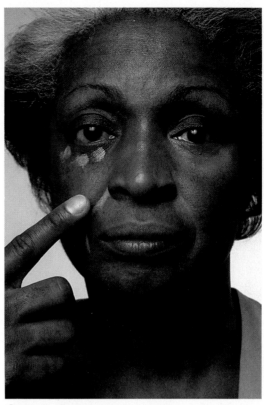

Step 2: Cover-up

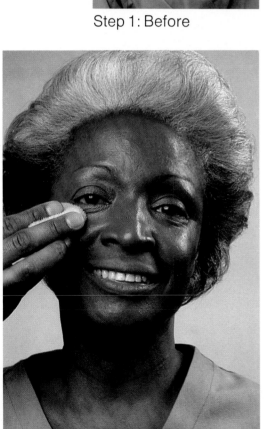

Step 3: Foundation

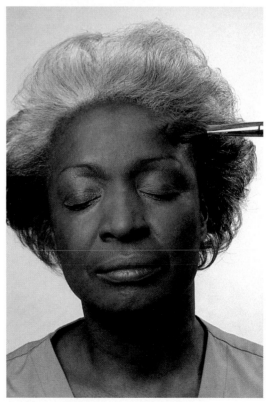

Step 4: Powder

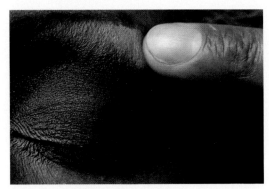

Step 5: Highlighter

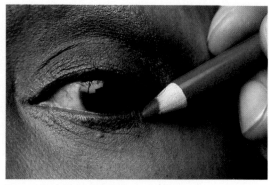

Step 6: Lining bottom rim

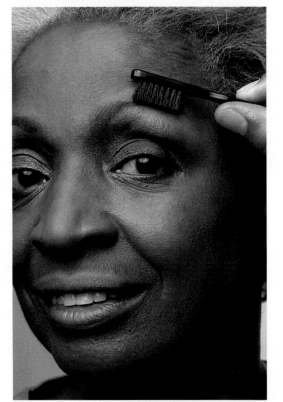

Step 7: Brushing up brows

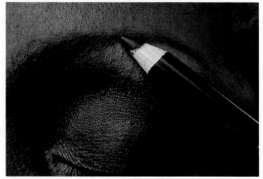

Step 8: Eyebrow pencil

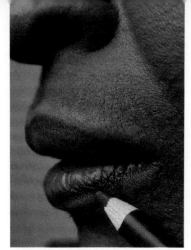

Step 9: Lip liner

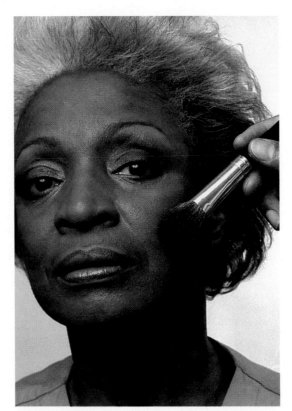

Step 10: Cheek blush

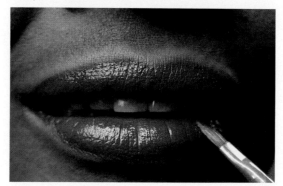

Step 11: Lip color with brush

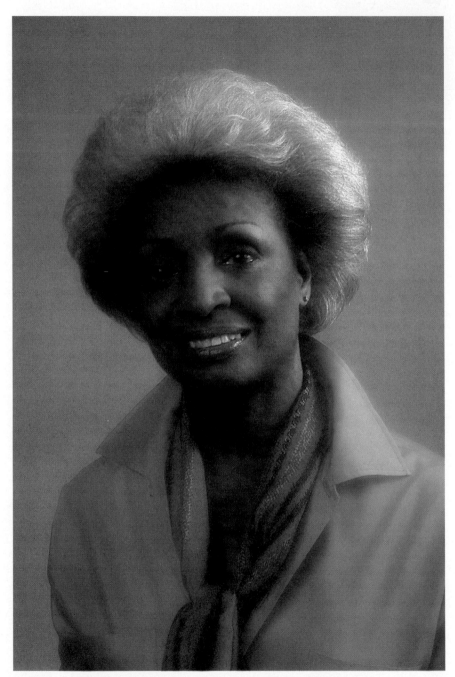

Step 12: After!

BEDTIME BRAIDS   Loosely braiding your hair at night and then pin-curling the braids (see page 25) will give you the softest, prettiest natural. It also adds length to your hair and will make it more manageable.

If your hair is very delicate and breaks easily, cover your hair with a silk, nylon, or smooth fabric scarf (never cotton) or sleep on nonabrasive pillow cases like satin or nylon.

The Art of Défrisage

Madame C. J. Walker gave us a new styling option when she invented the hot comb. This was the first time the tight curliness of our hair could be released, and a larger curl put back in by using a curling wand.

Madame Walker was born on December 23, 1867, in slavery in Louisiana (it did not rejoin the Union until 1868, three years after the Civil War had ended). She began her research in 1901 at the age of thirty-four, and when she died eighteen years later, she had the distinction of being America's first black millionairess.

Thermal-pressing and curling is still a popular method of temporarily relaxing the hair, allowing you to alternate with a natural. The choice is yours whenever you shampoo, and with new, modernized methods for pressing and curling, you can be assured that your hair will be both beautiful and fashionable.

A NEW NAME, TOO　A new technique deserves a name that reflects the effort, research, and skill involved in redevelopment. Innovative hairstylist Walter Fountaine popularized *défrisage* (a French word pronounced day-free-saje) which means simply to defrizz–the contemporary terminology for press and curl.

HAIR THAT BLOWS IN THE WIND　As its new name indicates, thermal-pressing has come a long way since its beginnings. Rose Morgan, proprietor of the House of Beauty in New York City and one of the pioneers in establishing quality salons for Black women, has the trademark of "hair that blows in the wind." Here are her directions for the new method of défrisage.

HOW TO DÉFRISAGE

Shampoo your hair, lathering twice with a cleansing shampoo to remove any residue of oil from your previous treatment. Apply conditioning shampoo for the third and final lather and rinse thoroughly.

Wrap your hair in a towel to blot the excess water. Massage ½ teaspoon of a very thin, lightweight oil between the palms of your hands and rub this into your hair while it is still wet. This will insure that your hair will dry with the oil absorbed into the hair shaft, protecting it from the heat without giving you a heavy, artificial sheen. You will not need to apply anymore oil to your hair. Comb through your hair with a pick or a wide-tooth comb.

Dry your hair using a blow-dryer with the setting on cool. Keep the dryer ten inches away from your hair. While hair is still slightly damp put the dryer down and gently comb through your hair with a wide-tooth comb. Continue to dry. This will remove most of the curl even before you press your hair. Comb through periodically to insure that all tangles are removed.

After your hair is completely dry, separate it into four sections—a center part from the crown to the nape of the neck, and a horizontal part from ear to ear. Roll and clip three of the sections out of the way. Use hand and wall mirrors so you can easily see the back and sides.

Now, you are ready to press your hair. Since most of the curl has been released as you were drying, it is not necessary to use a comb that is very hot. An electric heater is preferred to the kitchen jets because it's more sanitary. Always test your iron comb by wiping it on a clean towel or cloth. This also removes any oil from the hot comb.

As you comb through your hair, bend the comb so that the back of it is smoothed along the entire length of your hair; be careful not to touch your scalp with the comb. When you complete the first section, clip it out of the way and continue to the next one.

Once all hair is pressed, you are ready to curl it. You can use either an electric or standard iron curling wand. Electric ones are best because the heat is regulated. If you are using a standard wand, test it each time you remove it from the flame or electric heater to make another curl by clamping the curling wand around tissue paper.

Clip curls with bobby pins or metal clips until they cool.

Wash and towel dry hot comb and curling wand so that they are ready for your next use.

Set your hair in pin curls at night (see page 25) to keep your style between shampoos.

Relaxing Your Hair Permanently

•—•

Relaxing your hair permanently means you can swim, enjoy sports, or get caught in the rain and your hair will not revert to its natural wave pattern. With new, improved products available, hair that is permanently relaxed can look and feel natural, with healthy texture and bouncy body.

HOW DOES IT WORK? The relaxer actually changes the molecular arrangement of hair. Here's how: The cuticular scales on the outer layer of the hair shaft loosen and the relaxer penetrates into the inner, cortex layer where it reforms the polypeptide chains, placing them in a new, straighter relationship to each other. The relaxer contains less than 2 per cent of *sodium hydroxide,* or lye, which, to date, is the most effective ingredient on the market to relax hair.

To physically help the bonds reform, hair is smoothed with the back of a comb or rubber-gloved fingers during the application. Afterward, a *neutralizing* shampoo stops the action of the relaxer.

RELAXING AT HOME Your initial treatment should be done professionally so that you can consult your stylist about your hair's condition and get the personal advice and suggestions your hair deserves. Once your stylist has given you the O.K. to relax your hair at home, here are some guidelines.

WHEN NOT TO RELAX Your hair and scalp should be in optimum condition before you apply a relaxer. If your hair is damaged with broken, split ends, have a series of deep-conditioning treatments a month or so before you relax. If your scalp is irritated or scratched, do not relax your hair. First, see a dermatologist to solve the problem.

Shampooing opens your scalp's pores, making it susceptible to burn, so wait three days after your last shampoo to relax your hair. Wigs, hairpieces, cornrows, or anything that applies pressure or causes tension should be avoided before your treatment. Coffee dilates the blood vessels in your scalp, increasing the chances of irritation, so drink it after, not before, your relaxer.

If your hair is treated with any type of color or rinse, you should not apply a relaxer until three to four weeks after your color treatment. Never apply both on the same day, because mixing two chemicals puts too much stress on your hair and could result in breakage and hair loss.

RETOUCHING To keep your hair beautifully relaxed, it has to be retouched every six to eight weeks or when you have ½ inch of new growth. Don't wait too long though, because hair that is partially relaxed will snap easily where it goes from straight to curly. And don't relax *too often* or you will overlap and cause breakage. To make sure you are having regular treatments, keep an accurate record by marking your calendar.

Once you've had your first treatment, only the new growth of hair has to be retouched. If you retouch hair that has already been relaxed, it will become thin and fragmented because the same bonds are reformed again and again. Hair that is overlapped or overrelaxed looks frizzy and feels dry and brittle. Splitting and breakage are a major problem. *Only* apply the relaxer to your untreated hair.

MAINTAINING BEAUTIFUL TEXTURE For your hair to maintain its healthy texture, you should know which strength formula is right for you. How long you apply and smooth the relaxer is important, too, so that you can prevent having overrelaxed, dull, lifeless hair.

Always use a timer set for the *total* amount of minutes, and no matter what, don't exceed the recommended time. Leaving the relaxer on until the scalp burns causes *scarring alopecia*—a burned scalp resulting in irreversible hair loss.

	PRODUCT STRENGTH	TO APPLY	TO SMOOTH	TOTAL
FINE HAIR	Mild	3 minutes	5 minutes	8 minutes
MEDIUM HAIR	Regular	5 minutes	7 minutes	12 minutes
THICK HAIR	Strong	7 minutes	9 minutes	16 minutes

HOW TO APPLY A RELAXER

Ask a relative or a friend to help you. Be sure to have all your tools set aside: relaxer kit, rubber gloves, two towels (one for your hair and one to put around your shoulders), mirrors, tint brush, small-tooth comb, wide-tooth comb, timer, neutralizing shampoo, conditioner.

Read all the instructions in your kit carefully and be sure you understand everything before you begin. Take the phone off the hook.

To determine exactly how long you will need to relax your hair, do a strand patch test: Take a small section of hair from the side of your hair in the back where mistakes can be easily camouflaged. Apply the relaxer, following all of the steps. If you experience any discomfort or breakage, discontinue the treatment.

Do use a base, even if the product says it's not necessary. In this case, a petrolatum or wax base pomade is preferable. Apply it to your scalp in small sections, then gently massage it in to insure that your entire scalp is covered. Apply the pomade to the top and back of your ears and all around the edges of your hairline.

Part your hair into three sections. Begin your first part from ear to ear, across the top of your head. Part the larger back section into two by dividing from top to bottom in the middle. Secure the front and one back section out of your way.

Use wall and hand mirrors so you can clearly see the back, sides, and top of your hair.

Use a timer. Set it to the recommended total time before you begin the actual application of the relaxer.

Hair and scalp must be dry. Do not shampoo before you relax.

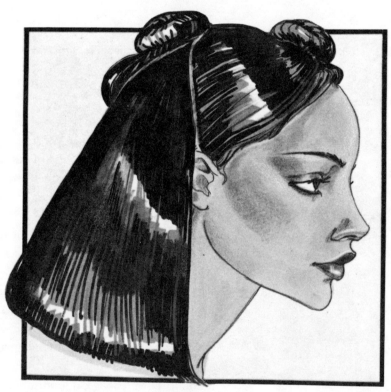

Using a tint brush or small-tooth comb for quick, even application, apply the relaxer to the top side of your hair, keeping the material off your scalp.

When applying it to the back section, place the treated hair toward the front. When applying it to the front section, place the treated hair over the back.

Apply the relaxer in the direction of hair growth. Since the ends are more porous and relax the easiest,

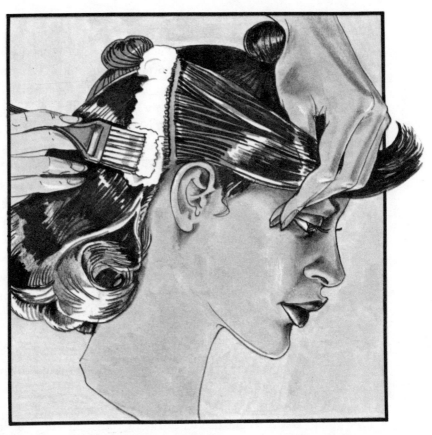

apply always from the scalp outward if you are
relaxing for the first time. If you are retouching,
apply only to new growth.

Once the relaxer is applied to the section, go back
to your starting point and smooth the relaxer with
quick, tiny strokes, top to bottom. Use the back of a
comb or the fleshy part of your rubber-gloved
fingertips. Be gentle. Your hair is extremely delicate
at this point.

When the timer goes off, thoroughly rinse the
relaxer immediately. Use warm water for at least five
minutes and don't forget to rinse the edges and parts
very well. Shampoo with the neutralizing shampoo to
halt the action of the relaxer. This should be
included in your kit.

Follow the same procedure for applying the relaxer
to the remaining sections, leaving the front for last.
(You may want to relax your hair in two sections
instead of three, treating the back as all one section.)

When you're finished, shampoo your hair again with the neutralizing shampoo. Three separate sudsings completely stop the relaxing action inside the cortex layer, so use all of your shampoo. Do not use a cleansing shampoo. Your neutralizing shampoo also cleans the pomade from your scalp.

Give yourself a wonderful, pampering conditioner with the conditioner contained in your kit. It should be especially designed as a postrelaxing conditioner to restore some of the moisture that's been lost and replace strength and elasticity. It will also restore natural oils. If your kit does not have a conditioner, see Bruce's treatment on page 38. Rinse thoroughly, combing through with a wide-tooth comb. Set hair as usual. Never blow-dry after a relaxing treatment.

THE WET SET After you relax and shampoo your hair, you are ready to set it on rollers. Once your hair has been relaxed, the only way to dry and set it is the wet set, because it is gentle for your hair. Blow-dryers and curling wands may be good for occasional use, but constant use will dry out your hair and will leave it looking dull and lifeless.

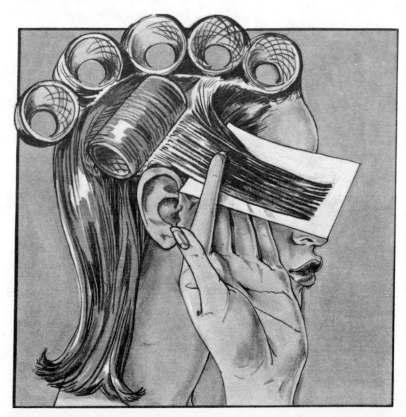

When you set your hair, the rollers should be firm, but not so tight that they pull or hurt your scalp. Smooth plastic rollers used with pointed metal hairclips are easiest to use at home because you don't need end papers. The more popular mesh rollers give a nice, firm set. You'll need end papers to keep the ends from getting frizzy. Again, never use sponge rollers.

Just before you are ready to set your hair, spray first with a cream rinse to make combing easier. Then, spray with a mixture of equal parts vinegar and water to help restore your hair back to normal pH level. An extra occasional spritz while you are setting will keep ends from frizzing.

Always dry your hair under a hooded dryer. The heat of the dryer reinforces the curl. Your hair dries quickly, locking in moisture in the hair shaft. The result: shinier-looking hair.

A mesh hairnet will keep the rollers in place until your hair dries. The heat of the dryer should feel comfortable, never too hot. Drying time varies depending on the length and thickness of your hair, as well as the size of the rollers you use. In general, thirty-five minutes to one hour is plenty.

THE COMB OUT   After your hair has dried, let the rollers cool completely before taking them out. If you're under the dryer, set it on cool for the final five minutes. Your set will last longer.

Brush through your hair once or twice with your plastic-bristled brush to get rid of any parts or separations. Then style with your comb, using a rattail to lift hair.

As often as you can, use your wide-tooth comb to comb and style your hair. It minimizes breakage from daily handling.

To maintain your style between shampoos, set at night with pin curls; follow directions on page 25.

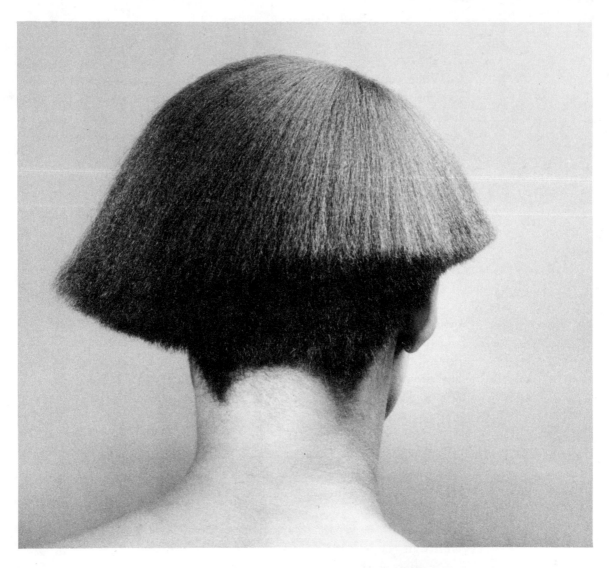

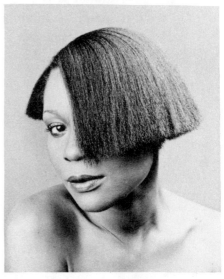

Afrology—New Wave of the Future

Increased awareness and new information have helped us to understand our hair's characteristics and appreciate its limitless possibilities. Hair can be partially relaxed and then reshaped into styles that transcend the traditional Anglo-Saxon definitions. Working with our hair's natural texture, we are exploring its unmeasured boundaries. The future holds exciting promises for us. Hair that's wash-and-wear is the ultimate in freedom.

SELECTIVE RELAXING   *Afrology,* a new styling concept by John Atchison of the John Atchison Salon in New York City, is a relaxed extension of the natural.

Using a relaxer, hair is selectively relaxed so that it still maintains most of it's natural texture. It is looser, with more movement.

Next, John, who apprenticed with master cutter Vidal Sassoon, sculpts and molds the hair through precision cutting. His hairstyle left is one example of how he uses geometric shapes to complement each woman's bone structure and features. Hair now functions on its own and never has to be set or curled.

THE THREE-WAY WET LOOK   Through selective relaxing, the natural experiences new dimensions, too. Dianne Turner calls this the Three-way Wet Look because by applying a relaxer for just a few minutes, you can wear your hair wavy, curly, or in a softly frizzed natural. Here are her directions for your at-home Afrology hairstyle.

HOW TO BEGIN
Shape your hair (see page 62) and lightly relax hair with a mild formula for a total of three to five minutes (see page 69). If hair is not relaxed enough, wait six to eight weeks before repeating treatment.

WET AND WAVY

Rub a small amount of a creamy liquid conditioner, lightweight oil, or setting gel between the palms of your hands and apply to wet hair. Comb your hair with a small-tooth comb, slightly weaving it in and out of your hair to create tiny little waves. Let dry.

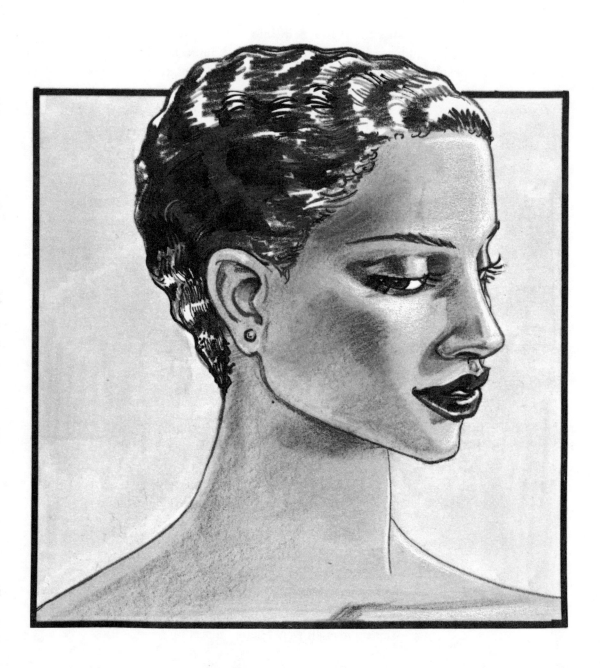

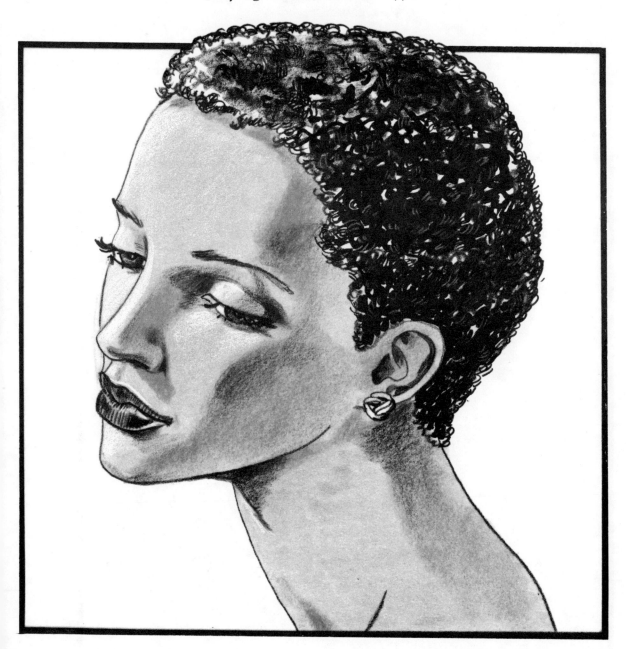

WET AND CURLY
Rub a small amount of a creamy liquid conditioner, lightweight oil, or setting gel between the palms of your hands and apply to wet hair. Pick out your hair, then fluff it a bit with your fingers. Let dry.

FRIZZED NATURAL
Pick your hair while it is still wet. Let dry almost
completely, then gently brush. Pick out again. Let
dry.

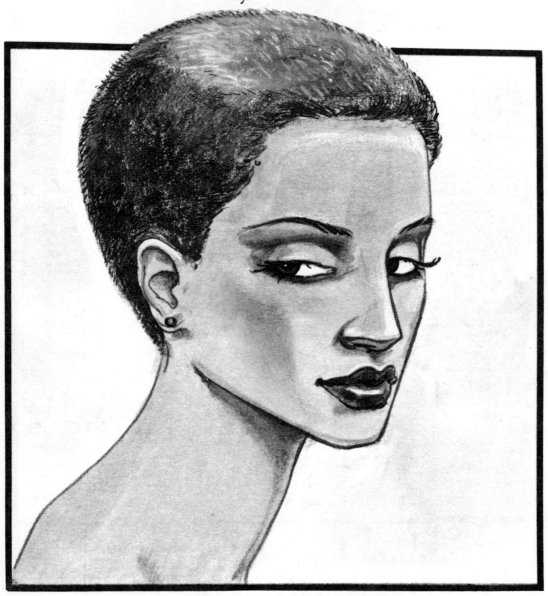

PERMANENT WAVES   In addition to relaxers, Walter Fountaine achieves
a similar effect by using permanent-wave solutions on virgin
hair to produce soft waves.

Permanent waving involves both chemical and physical operations that are the reverse of relaxing. An alkaline solution

changes the molecular structure of straight hair to curly. To physically help this change, hair is tightly wound on curlers called permanent-wave rods.

Caution: *Never* use a permanent-wave solution if your hair is relaxed.

REDIRECTING THE CURL According to Eric Turner, the solution to create large loose curls will neither a relaxer nor a permanent wave be, but rather a new, different product, yet to be developed, that actually combines both processes.

Relaxers take out the curl. Permanent waves make little waves. Neither makes a larger curl. This concept, called *redirecting the curl,* operates on the principle of taking our hair's natural curl and making it larger, softer.

FUNCTIONAL HAIR Eric, whose hairstyle is featured below, compares hair to a garment. Whether the material is wool, cotton, or silk

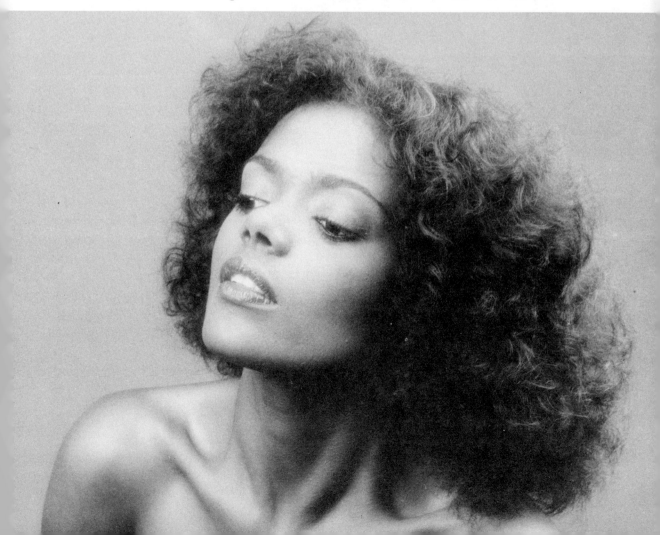

is unimportant as long as the clothes fit and complement your body. A blouse, for instance, continues to function for you even after you wash it. You do not have to sew the sleeves back in after it dries. He believes our hair has to function for us the same way. It should not have to be reshaped with rollers just because it's been washed.

A BREAKTHROUGH   A preview into the future promises development of a new, sophisticated technique that will be a breakthrough for Black hair. It will offer us yet *another* alternative: to redirect the natural curl in our hair to a larger curl, cultivating the strength and uniqueness of Black hair. Such a breakthrough is an idea whose time has come.

Cornrowing and Hairwrapping

Cornrowing and hairwrapping are exciting ways of adorning and decorating your hair. Intricate braid patterns and diagonal twists create long-lasting styles that are as practical as they are pretty.

FROM YESTERDAY TO TODAY   Cornrowing is an ancient African living art form. Even today, it's easy to identify an African woman's age, marital, and social status just by the way her hair is cornrowed.

This style is still very popular in contemporary hair fashions. In fact, once again Black women have set another trend. Couture designers have discovered this elegant, convenient way of hairstyling, and cornrows have now crossed ethnic lines. They can be seen on everyone—everywhere!

FROM WEDDING TO HONEYMOON   The bride who wants to combine both her African and American heritages is breathtaking in chiffon and pearled cornrows. Expert Sonia Bullock designed this hairstyle for *Bride's* magazine. Pearls are actually sewn in the very top layers of the braids. For everyday, she suggests adding beads, ribbons, or colorful cords as an extra, playful touch.

Because they last and last, cornrows for both natural and relaxed hair are especially perfect for honeymoons, long weekends, vacations—or anytime—when you want to spend your leisure hours doing everything but worrying about your hair. To keep the braids neat while you sleep, cover your hair with a silk or nylon scarf (cotton is too abrasive). Never brush your braids.

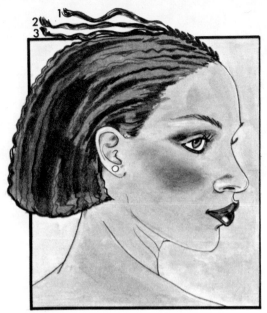

BRAIDING YOUR HAIR   Let a relative, friend, or your maid-of-honor braid your hair the day before the wedding. Set aside two hours to do it. First, wash and condition your hair. Blow-dry with the setting on cool, keeping the dryer ten inches away from your hair. Comb hair back. Starting at the top center of your hair, part a section from forehead to crown. Divide section into three hanks. Fold hank 1 over 2 then 3 over 1, while weaving in short strands from the scalp so the cornrow lies flat. When you reach the crown area, secure with a bobby pin.

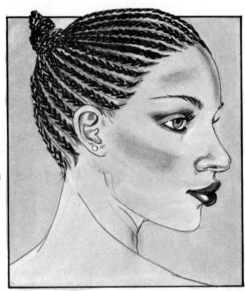

TYING A SMALL KNOT   Continue even sectioning and braiding all around your head, angling the cornrows toward the crown. Remove bobby pins and gather cornrow ends into a ponytail, and secure. Twist the ponytail into a knot. Pin. Then wrap a silk or nylon kerchief around your head so you can sleep without disturbing cornrows.

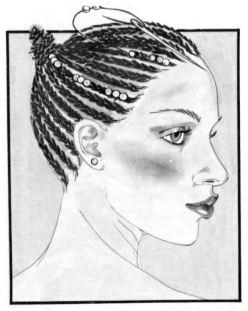

BEADING THE CORNROWS   Set aside two hours on wedding morning to do this. Thread a sewing needle with black thread (or thread to match the color of your hair); knot. Sewing away from your forehead, carefully glide needle into beginning of cornrow to anchor knot. Slide pearls or colorful beads (Sonia used three pearls) on needle. Weave needle in, then out; slide on more pearls. Leave an inch between each grouping. At the end of the row, knot and cut thread. Repeat, beading every fourth row. To remove beads, carefully lift thread, cut, pull out pearls or beads.

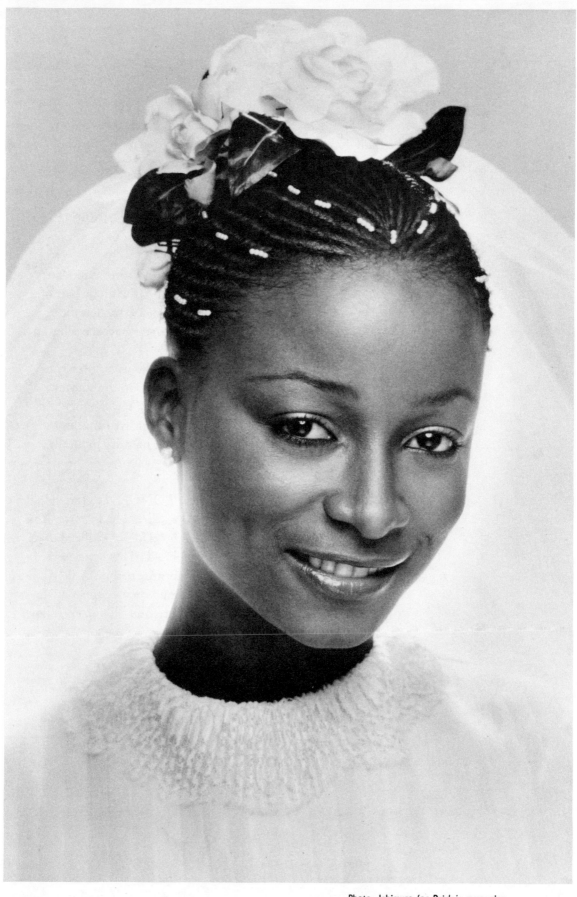

Photo: Ishimuro for *Bride's* magazine
Makeup: Byron Barnes

SUDS IN YOUR ROWS Your cornrow style can last as long as two weeks, and although *deep* cleaning your scalp is impossible to do while your hair is braided, you can shampoo to remove surface dust and dirt without ruining your hair. Here are Sonia's directions.

HOW TO SHAMPOO YOUR CORNROWED HAIR

Suds shampoo between the palms of your hands and massage it into your hair. Use only the fleshy part of your fingertips. Be very careful not to scratch the exposed scalp. Massage gently since vigorous rubbing will undo your braids.

Rinse thoroughly by running the water over your hair. You may find this easiest to do in the shower. Gently blot any excess water with a towel. Then, tie your hair with a soft fabric scarf for five minutes to "set" the cornrows flat again. Let hair dry naturally.

MAKING INDIVIDUAL BRAIDS LONGER, LONGEST Individual braids are braids that are not attached to the scalp in rows. You can make them as long as you like by adding artificial hair, called *extensions,* to your own as you braid. This style is versatile, too, because you can begin with cornrows, then make individual braids, or you can wear the braids loose one day and gathered in a ponytail the next. For care and shampoo, follow the same suggestions as for cornrows.

JUST A REMINDER Remember that wearing your hair braided too tightly, or for too long, will pull it right out of the scalp. You will lose all the lanugo hairs around the edges of your hairline. Cornrows are beautiful and fun, but they should be worn as alternatives to your everyday hairstyle.

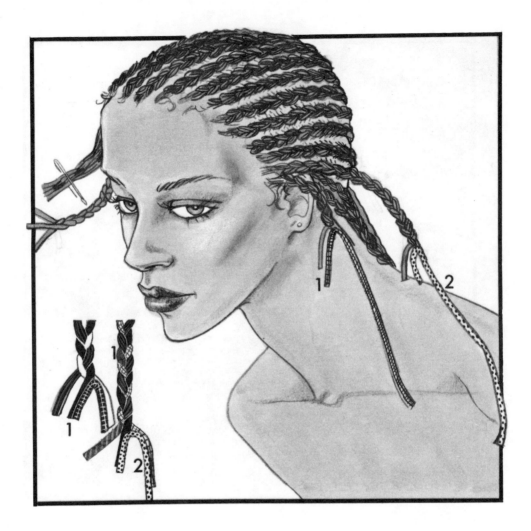

Sonia suggests you begin this style by cornrowing hair all back, toward the nape of the neck. (For how to cornrow, see directions for wedding braids.) To extend the braids, use artificial or human hair or "extensions" that match your own color and texture.

Begin by using an extension the thickness of one hank of hair. Bend the extension with the short end as the center hank and the long end blending in with your own hair. Braid until it's secure. Then add a second extension to another hank of your own hair; braid, and then add a third. Continue braiding until hair is the length you want. Trim the ends.

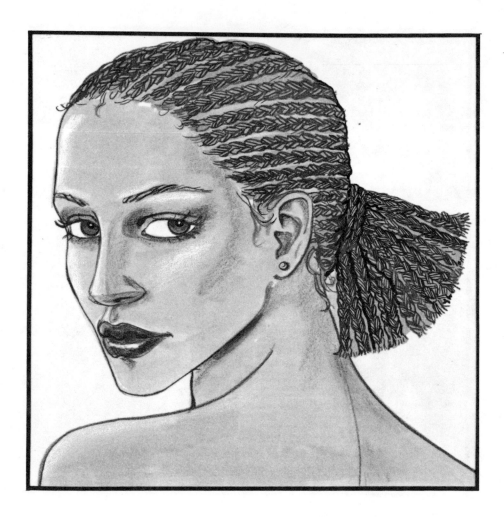

*Extensions look natural if you braid neatly and evenly.
This may take a little practice, so be patient. Once you
become adept, you can vary the styles, choosing more
intricate patterns. For individual braids that are not attached
to the scalp at all, add all three extensions as close to the
scalp as possible.*

FAST, FAT BRAIDS The larger your braid, the less likely you are to pull
your hair too tightly. The cornrow that goes from one side of
your head to the other is elegant and fashionable, perfect for
evening as well as daytime wear.

Plaits are braided with an inward motion and are flat braids that are closer to the scalp. The *French Braid* is braided with an outward motion and is raised so that you can see the entire design of the braid. Sonia prefers the French Braid for mature women, and suggests this is more flattering than lots of tiny cornrows. You can achieve the same effect by combing all hair off the face and adding an artificial braid. Tuck the ends of your hair under the braid.

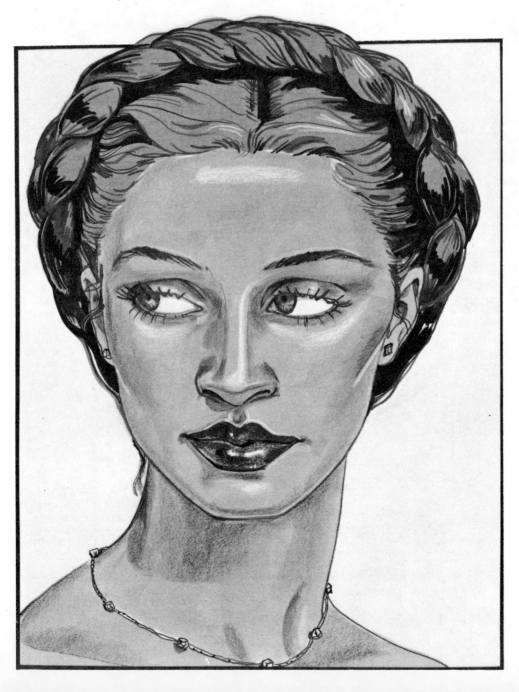

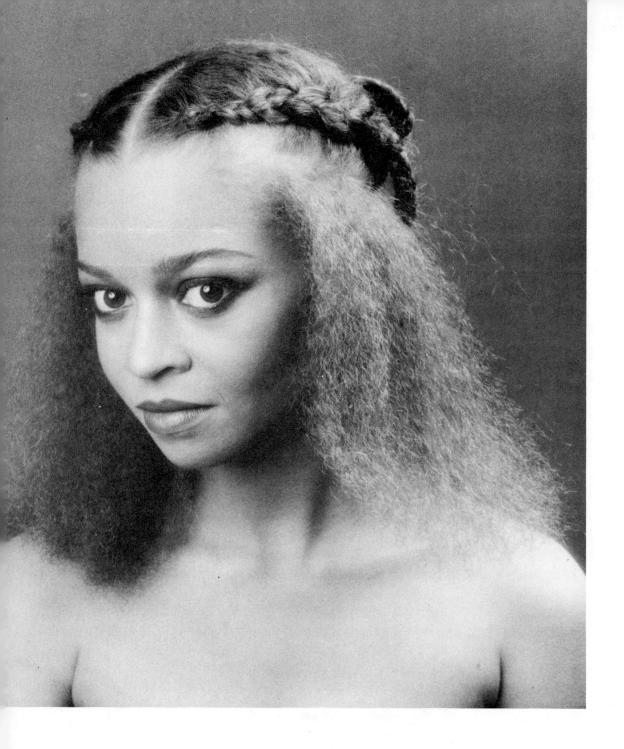

Sonia's protégée, Diane Law, created this style, called "The Butterfly," for long hair. For softness, leave a crimped row of loose hair to frame your face and neck. Then French-braid, tying the ends in the back to form a butterfly-type bow. To help bend the braids so they are elevated, take a hairpin, open it, and weave it in and out of the braids.

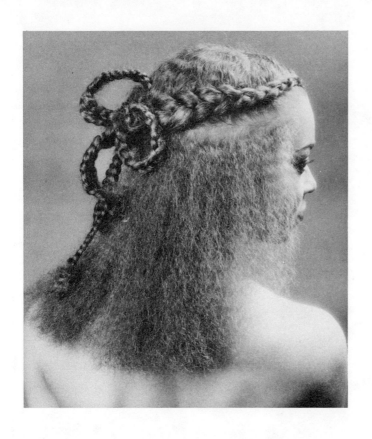

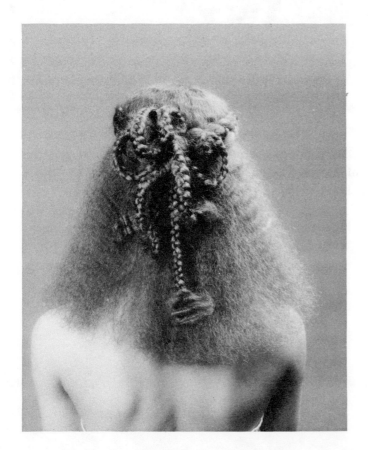

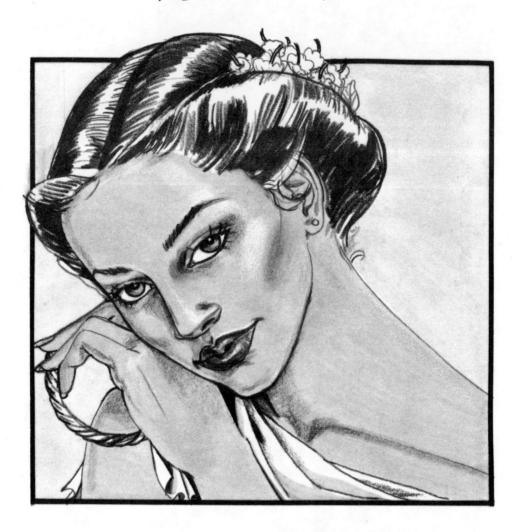

WRAPPING IT UP Hairwrapping, a rebirth of the forties' hairdo, is the most contemporary adaptation of African cornrowing. Since hours of braiding can be reduced to minutes with twists and face-framing rolls, hairwrapping reflects the fast pace of our changing lifestyle.

TWISTING IT TOGETHER The principle of hairwrapping is exactly the same as in cornrowing. Each section of hair is lifted and weaved into the hair preceding it, forming a ropelike effect. Hairpins or bobby pins anchor the rolled hair, keeping it firm and in place.

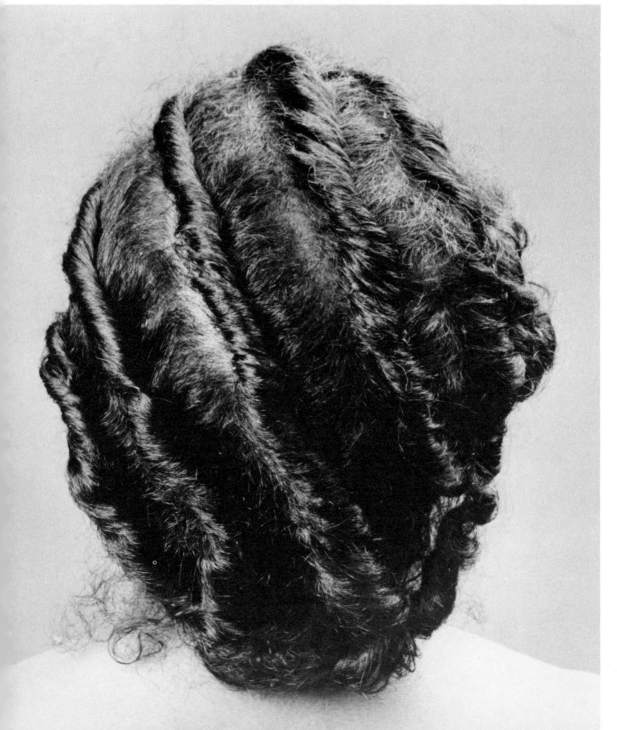

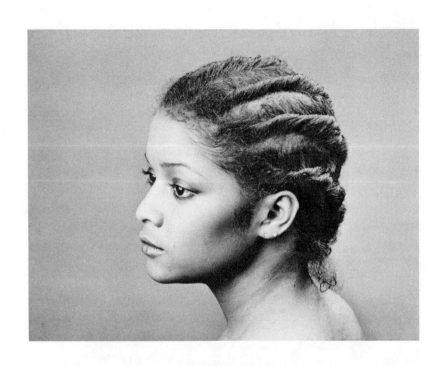

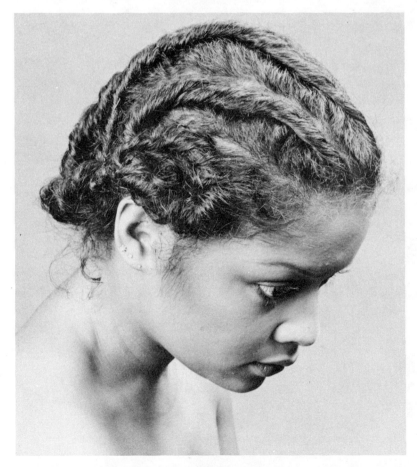

Hairwrapping can be as versatile as your imagination will allow. You can create exotic, diagonal twists in patterns very similar to cornrows, as Eric Turner illustrates. Just part and twist from top to bottom, pinning with hairpins where necessary. Once the roll is complete, secure the bottom with a bobby pin. Then continue on to the next section, repeating as before until all your hair is wrapped. Remove the pins and twist the bottom sections together or leave the wisps loose for a more dramatic effect.

Eric also recommends twisting your hair while it's wet, following your shampoo. This is great for appliance-free vacations, because your hair is immediately wearable—no dryers, no rollers. And when you comb your hair out, you will have softly crimped waves.

You can wrap all of your hair or just part of it. Also, a wonderful variation for the long natural is to roll the top section back and off the face—a welcome relief for hot summer days.

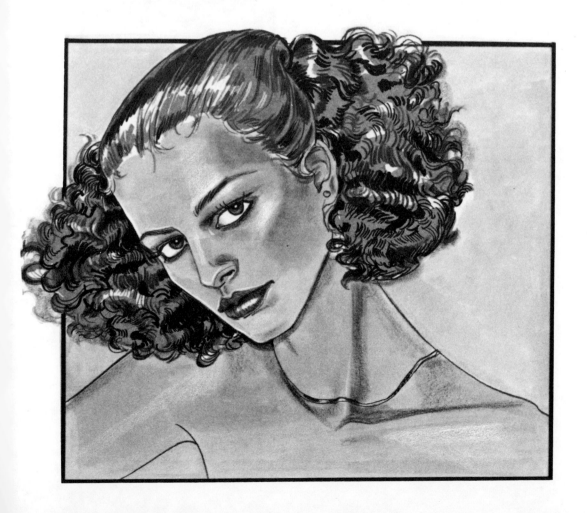

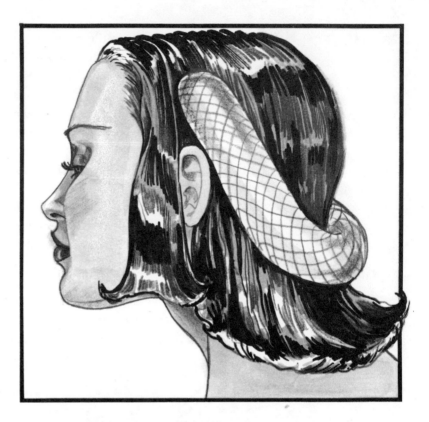

FILLING IT IN The larger roll is probably the most popular and the most formal of hairwrapping styles. Long hair can easily be rolled up while shorter hair achieves the same effect with just a little help.

The illustrations show how to comb your hair to attach a *filler*. You can purchase a ready-made one from department or wig stores. Or improvise your own. A false braid or hairpiece can be an ideal filler. Attach to your hair with bobby pins, then roll your own hair around this, tucking ends around filler. Secure with hairpins or bobby pins.

Dress up the final look by adding decorated combs, beads, or pearls. For an authentic African touch, sew a colorful cord right into the roll itself, as illustrated by Frenchie right.

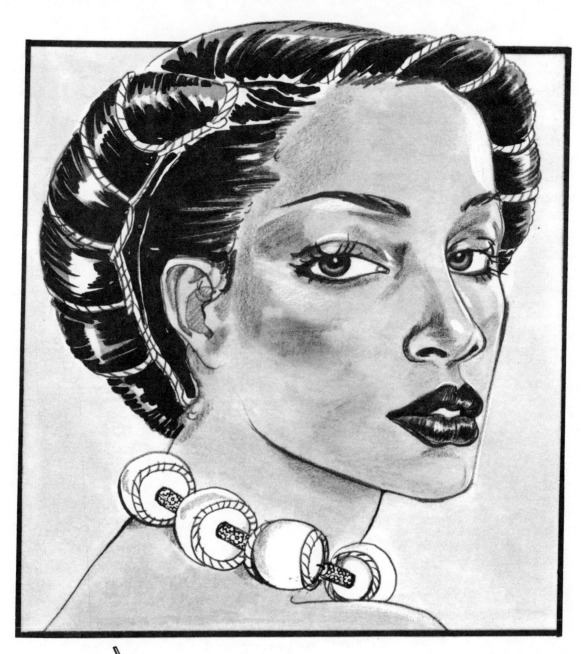

This stitched piece of fabric shows you how to sew the colorful cord around your rolled hair.

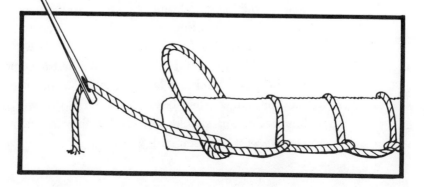

Wigs—a Beauty Wardrobe Basic

— • — • — • — • — • — • — • — • — • — • — • — • — • — • — • — • —

Your beauty wardrobe is not complete without a good-quality wig. It's an accessory that's versatile, fun, and carefree, allowing you to change your look whenever you want to.

Business trips and vacations are times in particular when you want to be fabulously flexible. And having the ultimate accessory that feels comfortable and looks as natural as if it were your own is the result of careful buying, handling, and care.

YOUR FIRST WIG   Your first wig should be very close to your own hair color and style, advises talented designer André Douglas of "It's a Wig!" And it should complement your features, personality, and lifestyle.

Choosing a curly wig means you can experiment with a lighter color. A straight texture requires a color that closely matches your own because it must blend in with your hair at the hairline.

If your hair is gray, choose shades that are slightly lighter than your own hair used to be. Wearing colors that are too dark, such as black, accentuates tiny lines and wrinkles.

Wigs range in texture from synthetic fibers to human hair. Synthetic fibers are longer lasting because they can be shampooed without losing their curl.

A COMFORTABLE CAP   It's very important that the cap on your wig be as sheer and lightweight as possible. This allows your scalp to breathe and eliminates pressure at the hairline where your own hair is the most delicate. In fact, André stresses that all the edges of your hairline be free. The wig cap should actually be a few inches back from your hairline. Avoid wigs that have ear tabs; they will rub and cause your own hair to come out.

The cap should also be stretchable so that it easily adjusts to the contour of your head. Always try the wig on before you buy because it should feel comfortable immediately. You cannot expect it to loosen with wear.

PERSONALIZING YOUR WIG   If you purchase a wig and find the style too full or too long, then it's probably not your style. Try to find a similar wig that is a bit shorter, for instance.

André advises that wigs are generally precision cut in the factory, and if you find you need to cut your wig once you get it home, remember that you are actually altering the natural wig style. Usually some of the curl is cut off, and it's impossible to put that curl back. You may curl it temporarily, but it probably will not last.

Geometric shapes often have to be trimmed and are usually designed longer for this reason. Have this done by your hairstylist, though, because it's too easy to make a mistake and ruin your new wig.

THE TRICK IS TO BLEND   You can easily camouflage the hairline of your wig by placing it *behind* your own hairline when you put it on. Comb and blend your own hair into the wig's.

If you prefer hair on your forehead, comb the hair from the wig onto your forehead but never pull the entire cap down so that it fits like a hat.

Before you put on your wig, protect your own hair by neatly wrapping or braiding it and covering it with a hairnet. If your hair is very long, part it in the middle and, bringing each section forward from the back to the front, wrap the sections around your head and secure with hairpins or bobby pins.

If your hair is short or medium length, pin curls (see page 25) will keep it from bulging underneath. If you are wearing a natural, braid or cornrow your hair (see page 82).

For swimming and active sports, be sure to secure the wig firmly with bobby pins that are the same color as your wig hair.

BRUSH YOUR WIG   It's important to brush your wig often, especially at the nape area. After a period of time, wear and perspiration remove the protective coating from the hair, causing it to frizz. Brush in a small amount of a lightweight oil to restore the sheen and texture.

A nylon brush with a rubber cushion is best for your wigs. Clean wig brushes frequently.

SHAMPOO IT TOO   Shampooing your wig keeps it fresh and attractive. A mild shampoo is best. Fabric softeners leave the hair too soft to hold the curl. Never comb or brush your wig while it is wet. Here are more of André's directions.

HOW TO SHAMPOO YOUR WIG

Always check the wig-care instructions before you shampoo.

For long or sleek styles, prepare two basins, one with warm shampoo water and the other with cool water for rinsing. Dip your wig in and out of the shampoo water. Rinse by dipping it in and out of the rinse water.

Dry the cap first by turning it inside out and setting it, cap up, under a cool dryer. You do not want to expose the hair unless you are setting it with rollers. Once the cap dries, turn the wig right side out and hang it on a hanger, securing with safety pins.

To shampoo short, curly, and frizzy styles, shampoo in warm water as above. To rinse, let cool water run through the curls. (Hot water will remove the curl.) To dry, you can hang it on a hanger immediately. Since the hair is short, both hair and cap will dry quickly.

THE RIGHT WAY TO STORE   The correct way to store your wig is by placing it on a wig head. If you store your wig in a box, you may fold it differently than when it was packed, creasing and altering the curl. For travel, just fold your wig inside out.

See page 164 for Andre's wig designs.

Skin
Care

Happy Skin

• — •

Skin that is nourished from the inside with the proper foods and kept balanced on the outside with a thorough cleansing program is not only beautiful, it's happy! And a clear, healthy, radiant complexion is your reward.

Maintaining skin that is lovely to look at from across a desk, or beautiful to touch at a candlelit table, says you care about yourself. It means you are intelligently utilizing all your beauty options to be the best woman you can possibly be—inside and out.

But skin is more than just a pretty face and body. It is your personal alarm system. It will loudly broadcast mistreatment through abuse from alcohol, cigarettes, and sun, by looking drawn, discolored, and aged. Excesses are not good for the spirit either, and there's a lot to be said for "clean" living when you see the results in your face as well as in your overall quality of life.

Your skin often alerts you to certain illnesses, allergies, or systemic disorders that might otherwise be overlooked. In this section, dermatologists offer basic guidelines and suggestions to help you listen and tune in to your body.

Clear skin forms the perfect palette for makeup. If you prefer to wear a minimal amount of makeup, or none at all, then your beauty regimen must be so well designed that your complexion is always flawless. The skin-care experts' advice will help you develop a simple yet effective lifetime beauty regimen.

As in the field of hair care, skin care has it's own myth to discard. A noted cosmetic surgeon, after years of research discovers and reveals how it is now possible for any Black woman to experience the luxury of cosmetic surgery.

Total skin care involves pampering all of you. Consistency is the key in keeping your face supple, your hands, feet, and body smooth. Happily, the beauty news here supports what we have always instinctively known. Black skin *is* truly beautiful skin. With the proper care and treatment, it will stay even younger looking longer.

Melanin, the Biggest Beauty Bonus

- -

Melanin, or pigment, is what gives us our warm kaleidoscope of colors. It is one of our biggest beauty bonuses. Melanin protects our skin from the harmful rays of the sun that cause aging and skin cancer.

Before we fully explore this particular phenomenon though, let's examine the complete anatomy of our skin.

BENEATH THE SURFACE   On the surface, skin shields the delicate inner organs and is the body's natural protection against the elements in our environment. It's the vehicle through which we experience sensations such as pleasure, pain, heat, and cold.

Beneath the surface, skin eliminates wastes from the body and, with the help of the circulatory system, transmits vital nutrients to both hair and nails.

Skin has three main sections—the epidermis, the dermis, and the hypodermis. The *epidermis* is the outer layer of skin and is itself comprised of three layers.

The top, or *horny*, layer is called the *stratum corneum* and is the visible portion of the skin. Here, skin acts as a buffer, catching environmental impurities and reacting to temperature and humidity changes. To renew itself, the stratum corneum constantly sheds old skin every twenty-seven days. This process is called *exfoliation*, or the sloughing off of dead skin cells.

Fresh new cells are replenished from the *basal* layer which is the innermost layer of the epidermis. The middle layer is where the hair follicles are and is called the *stratum granulosum.*

Below the epidermis is the *dermis.* Here, *sudoriferous,* or sweat, glands modulate body temperature. When the body is overheated or under stress, these sudoriferous glands serve as ventilation, carrying perspiration to the surface to cool the body. Contrary to popular myth, black skins contain the same number of sweat glands as do white skins.

The dermis contains other important glands, too. These are the *sebaceous* glands which secrete *sebum* or oil to lubricate the skin. Black skins do not have more sebaceous glands than white skins.

The last layer of skin, the *hypodermis,* contains fatty tissue which connects the skin to the bones and muscles. This tissue contains collagen or protein which is responsible for the elasticity of skin. The loss of this elasticity due to the aging process or excessive sun exposure results in taut skin and facial wrinkles.

ABSORBING THE LIGHT   The color of skin is the result of the reflection of light on its surface. When light hits our skin, our eye converts this reflection into a color.

Black skin absorbs the light. White skin reflects almost all light. What we see as the difference in skin colorations is actually the difference in light absorption.

But what determines the intensity of light absorption, giving us a myriad of complexion ranges from pale caramel to deep chocolate? Why do some black skins absorb more light than others?

MELANIN IS THE ANSWER   The answer is a tiny, light-brown substance called pigment, or melanin. The darker your skin color, the more melanin you have and the more light your skin absorbs.

Melanin is the body's protective shield against the sun's harmful rays. It prevents the toxic rays from penetrating to the basal layer of the epidermis where skin cancer develops and to the elastic tissues in the dermis where wrinkling takes place.

MAKING MELANIN   How does the body produce melanin? Where does it come from?

In the basal layer, there are cells called *melanocytes.* Everyone, regardless of their ethnic group, has the same amount of these cells.

In white skins, each melanocyte produces about one hundred tiny black grains called *melanosomes*. In black skin, melanocytes also produce melanosomes, but they are not tiny. Each one is approximately *four* times larger than the melanosomes in white skin.

JOURNEY TO THE TOP *Keratinocytes* are the cells that travel from the basal layer to the horny layer every twenty-seven days. In their journey to the top, keratinocytes transfer melanin.

In white skins, keratinocytes gather a bundle of melanosomes but along the way, the melanosomes completely disintegrate. When the keratinocyte reaches the stratum corneum, there are no pigment cells left.

However, in our skin, because the melanosomes are larger, the keratinocytes take fewer. As they move up to the top layer, they settle, becoming part of skin cells.

This entire process of making and transferring melanin is called *pigmentogenesis* and is determined by the genetic factor.

SENDING FOR HELP According to Dr. John A. Kenney, Jr., professor and chairman of the Department of Dermatology, Howard University College of Medicine, the production of melanin also occurs when your skin responds to injury, trauma, or exposure to the sun. Sometimes in an effort to send help, too much melanin is produced and dark spots, or *hyperpigmentation*, results.

Our skin produces melanin easily, and it hyperpigments easily too. Simply squeezing a pimple can cause hyperpigmentation. Sometimes, even if you don't squeeze a pimple can leave a temporary dark spot. Allergies to cosmetics and perfumes, or reactions to internal medications such as the birth-control pill, can also cause unattractive dark spots, Dr. Kenney explained.

In most cases, hyperpigmentation is only temporary and dark spots will gradually clear by themselves. Over-the-counter products containing at least 2 per cent of hydroquinone—a safe bleach used in skin creams to help lighten dark spots—can be effective in treating minor cases. However, if hyperpigmentation presents a major cosmetic concern, dermatologists often prescribe creams with a higher percentage of hydroquinone to quickly balance the complexion again. When using these products, it's important to limit sun exposure to discourage additional stimulation of pigment cells.

THE HORMONAL WHIP *Postinflammatory hyperpigmentation* is increased pigment that results from inflammation or irritation. This can occur if a pimple is improperly squeezed, spreading the foreign material back underneath the skin and causing the area to become inflamed and dark.

Postinflammatory hyperpigmentation presents a major concern for Black women who have acne. Although many factors cause acne, the most important factor is what Dr. Kenney describes as the hormonal whip.

Male hormones secreted by the ovaries and the adrenal glands encourage or "whip" the sebaceous glands to produce more and more oil. This overproduction initially results in small pimples such as whiteheads (closed comedones) or blackheads (open comedones).

It's important to stress here that not every whitehead or blackhead is acne. Blackheads can be due to oil that is trapped in your skin. It dries and hardens, clogging and enlarging the pore openings. The portion of dried sebum on the skin's surface becomes dark and this is why it is called a blackhead, or in medical terms, an *open comedone*.

A whitehead can also be caused by oil trapped beneath the surface of the skin. When it is opened, which because of the risk of hyperpigmentation, should only be done by a dermatologist or skin-care specialist, the oil that comes out is hard and white. The *closed comedone* must be squeezed to release the trapped oil. Whiteheads do appear in dry skins, too, and can be due to poor functioning of the oil glands. Skin massage is one way to correct the malfunction of these glands.

Acne occurs when the overproduction of oil continues until pus collects in the pimple and it becomes infected. At this stage they are called *papules* and are very tender and easily inflamed. If infected, the next stage is called *pustule,* and this is a severe case of acne.

Over-the-counter products containing *benzoyl peroxide* are the most effective in destroying bacteria that spread new acne infections. They may leave a whitish residue on dark skin, but this can be camouflaged with a sheer layer of water-based makeup. If you have acne, check with your doctor before using *any* makeup.

Even after acne has cleared, it often leaves temporary, sometimes permanent, hyperpigmentation resulting from the prolonged stress on the skin. Dr. Kenney recommends an opaque, waterproof concealing makeup that effectively evens the complexion, Covermark by Lydia O'Leary.

TURNING RED   Another type of pigment change is *erythema,* or a red spot. In our skin, erythema does not look red, but deep, dark purple. It can suggest an internal illness and should immediately be checked by a physician or dermatologist.

THE ABSENCE OF PIGMENT   Vitiligo is the result of *hypopigmentation.* Where pigment cells have actually been destroyed, areas on the skin are marked by an absence of pigment or color.

Although vitiligo occurs in other ethnic groups, it presents a significant cosmetic problem in black skins. Large areas of the skin are marked by white spots, which, though not visible in white skin, are strikingly evident in dark complexions.

Dr. Kenney, world renowned for his research and treatment of vitiligo, stimulates the production of pigment cells with Psoralin drugs. In cases where 50 per cent or more of the natural pigment is gone, Dr. Kenney removes the remaining pigment altogether so the complexion becomes one color.

Covermark is also very effective in masking the hypopigmented areas of vitiligo.

The Right Care for Delicate Skin

Keeping delicate skin smooth and healthy-looking requires just the right kind of care. And no package is as fragile or deserves more careful handling than your face.

All it takes is a few extra precautions to avoid premature wrinkling of your skin. Add easy, basic techniques to help you keep your face supple and smooth, and your skin will always feel as young as it looks.

TAKE IT OFF   To keep your skin radiant, take the extra few minutes to cleanse your face, no matter how tired you are in the evening. Makeup left on overnight seeps deep into your skin, clogging and enlarging your pores.

Sleeping with your mascara on guarantees you of losing at least four eyelashes each night. Remove your eye makeup with cleansing creams, makeup remover pads, or mineral oil.

THE HEADREST   When you're sitting at a table or desk, avoid that comfortable position of putting your elbows up and using your hands as a headrest. Your palms actually pull and stretch your skin, weakening the tissues around your mouth, cheeks, and neck. Whenever you rest your head in the palms of your hands, remember too, that you are actually transferring soil from your hands to your face.

In general, keep your hands away from your face altogether. You only need to touch your face when you are cleansing or applying makeup.

FACIAL EXPRESSIONS   Express yourself, but not with your face. Constant frowning, besides being an unpleasant facial expression, causes deep furrows in your forehead.

Squinting from the sun also causes wrinkles. Invest in a comfortable pair of lightweight sunglasses.

GOING IN CIRCLES   Applying soaps, creams, and lotions in upward, outward circular motions also retards wrinkles. You want every action, every application to help lift your face away from the pull of gravity.

Apply creams and lotions with cotton. It's gentle on delicate skin. You'll find rolls of nonsterile cotton easier to work with and more economical than cotton balls.

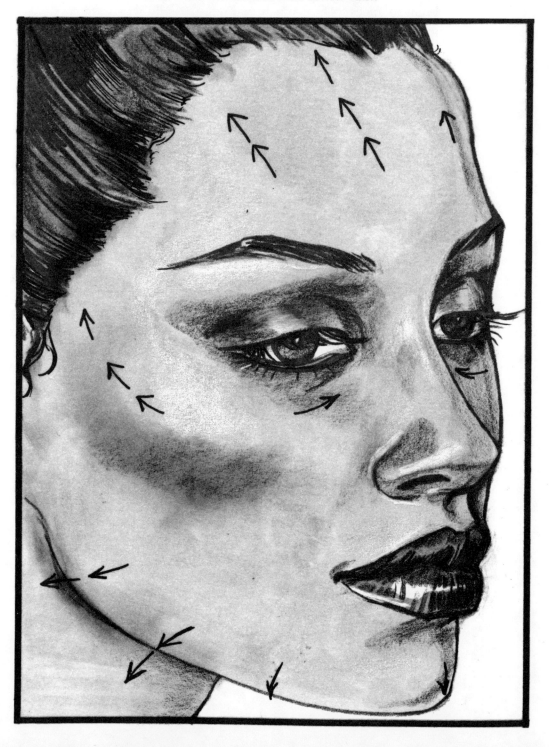

The skin around your eyes, especially underneath, is particularly fragile. Here, skin is thinner than on other areas of your face, and there are very few oil glands to hold the moisture. Eye creams, like moisturizers, are *humectants*. They draw and retain moisture and should be used by everyone—before lines begin to appear. Once you have lines, the only way to remove them is through cosmetic surgery.

Always apply your eye cream inward beginning at the outer edge of your eye and gently patting toward your nose (see arrows). Stretching and pulling outward toward the hairline encourages tiny fine lines called *crow's-feet*. Once you've applied the cream, blot the excess with tissue.

SMOOTHING THE SURFACE   Review how your skin replenishes itself. It's those tiny, exfoliated cells, more obvious on dark skin since the dead cells are white, that make skin look dry and feel rough.

Epiabrasion is the physical abrasion of the epidermis. It's one of the best ways to smooth the surface, removing oils and trapped impurities to leave your face and body with a clear, healthy glow. A loofah or a slightly abrasive synthetic sponge are two choice's for gently scrubbing away dead skin cells while stimulating circulation.

As much as possible, avoid using washcloths to clean or epiabrade your skin unless they are fresh from the laundry. Then, only use once.

Here's why: After you use a washcloth, it dries in the open, accumulating dust, dirt, and germs. Using it again puts these impurities right back onto your skin.

If you feel you need a cloth of some type to clean your face, take a fresh, large piece of cotton and wrap a paper towel around it. It's soft, yet abrasive, and after you finish just throw it away.

For a penetrating epiabrasion, use cleansing grains mixed with warm water to form a thin past. You can purchase them when you buy your cosmetics, or try uncooked oatmeal as a substitute. Gently massage your cheeks, chin, and forehead, avoiding the delicate area around your eyes. Since the grains are already abrasive, it's not necessary to scrub vigorously. Rinse thoroughly with warm water; repeat with cool. Use your cleansing grains only once or twice a week.

If your skin is in any way broken out or infected, do not use cleansing grains. You can easily spread infection to all areas of your face.

GETTING TO THE ROOT   Smoothing the surface also means getting rid of unwanted facial hairs above the lip or on the chin. Tweezing is usually painstaking and not very long-lasting. To remove hairs from your face permanently, you have to get to the root.

Waxing is one of the easiest, most effective ways to remove facial hairs. It removes the hair shaft and root totally and can be done on any part of the body. Regrowth is slow, and new hair is finer and thinner in texture. Over a period of time, the hair follicle is eventually destroyed and the hairs do not grow back at all.

If you follow the instructions on your waxing kit to the letter, waxing is easy to do at home. Apply warmed beeswax to your skin with a wooden spatula in the direction of hair growth. Place a strip of muslin on top of the warm wax. When the wax has cooled, which only takes a few seconds, quickly pull the cloth away against the hair growth.

DEPILATRON AND ELECTROLYSIS   Permanent methods of hair removal include *depilatron* and *electrolysis*. Both require a series of repeated treatments depending on your hair growth.

To remove hair through depilatron, an electronic tweezer sends heat currents deep into the hair follicle, sterilizing the papilla to prevent future hair growth. Hair grows back finer until the root is completely destroyed. This procedure is reportedly painless.

With electrolysis, a needle is inserted into the hair follicle orifice, sending sharp electrical currents to the root of each hair. Electrolysis is often painful and can leave areas of hyperpigmentation on black skin. It should only be administered by a trained, licensed electrologist.

BLEACHING   Bleaching is an effective way to camouflage facial hairs. Using only a product specifically designed for facial hairs, bleach your hair slowly, in stages, until the hairs are light enough to blend in with the color of your skin. This is particularly effective above the chin area and along the sides of the face.

Your Daily Cleansing Regimen

You *can* improve on a good thing. You can make your complexion lovelier by beginning where it counts, and that's with an effective daily cleansing regimen.

We have already seen how much wear and tear there is on the epidermis. Your face is constantly exposed, and dirt and pollution settle on the surface and seep into your pores. Only a well-thought-out beauty plan can give you deep-down clean skin that lets your natural beauty show through.

SMART SKIN CARE   Smart skin care begins while you're young and starts with a skin-care specialist to analyze your particular skin type. Or, a cosmetician in a department store can help you select products and treatments that are right for you. Problem skin, of course, requires the expertise of a dermatologist.

Check the product's consistency. Lightweight creams and lotions will give you the best results. Thick, petrolatum-based substances will clog your pores and irritate your skin.

KNOW YOUR SKIN TYPE   There are three basic skin types: normal, or combination, oily, and dry. Since the light reflected from dark skin makes it appear shiny, there is often confusion in identifying skin types. Shine does not mean that your complexion is oily. This simple tissue test eliminates the guesswork in identifying your skin type.

THE TISSUE TEST   In the morning, cleanse your face. Rinse very well. Do not apply lotion, moisturizer, or makeup.

After you've been fairly active, check your face around midday. Using just one layer of tissue, press it flat against your cheeks, chin, nose, and forehead. Examine the tissue in a good light and take a close look at your skin.

NORMAL/COMBINATION   If the tissue comes away from your face relatively clean, then yours is *normal* skin. Your face has a fresh appearance even in the middle of an active day.

However, the tissue may not be as easily removed from your chin, nose, and forehead as it is from your cheeks. When you examine it in the light, you see oily spots which are not in the cheek area.

On closer examination, the pores in this area, called the *T-zone,* may be slightly enlarged. Yours is *combination* skin. Your face is basically normal, but the T-zone is oily. Most women fall into this category, and it means you must pay extra attention to your T-zone to help balance your complexion.

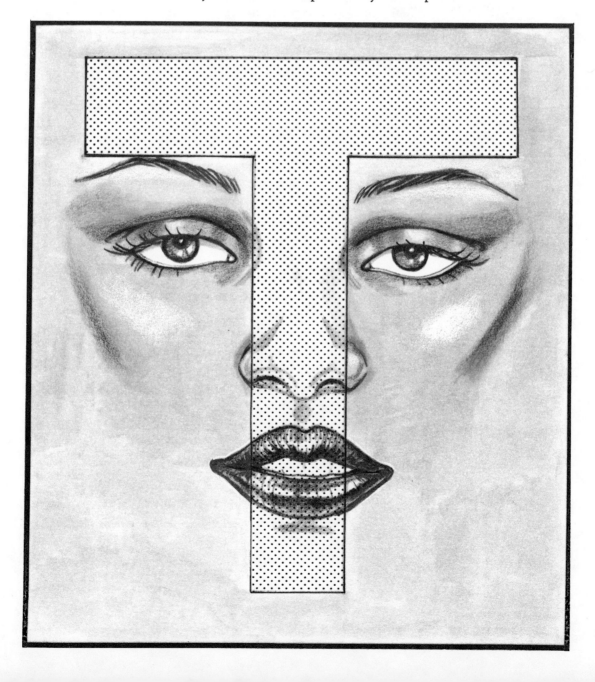

OILY SKIN   When you press the tissue to your face, it adheres quite easily, sticking, in fact. When you pull it away and examine it in the light, you can see that there are many oily spots. The pores on your entire face are enlarged. After an active morning, nothing would make you feel better than cleansing your face again.

Your skin type is *oily,* and you must balance your complexion to discourage whiteheads and blackheads that result from overproductive glands.

DRY SKIN   When you press the tissue to your face, it does not stick at all. Your face feels taut, without elasticity, and you see tiny flakes. You may even notice tiny, fine lines around your eyes and mouth.

Dry skin is the result of dehydration and underfunctioning sebaceous glands. Your beauty regimen should be designed to restore moisture to your skin.

A.M./P.M.   Maintaining and balancing your skin is something you do every day when you cleanse your face in the morning *and* at night. The daily regimen below is designed for your individual skin type. If your skin tends to be dry or sensitive you may want to use creamy cleansers instead of soaps.

DAILY REGIMEN FOR NORMAL/COMBINATION SKIN

Your morning cleansing begins with a mild glycerin soap, superfatted soap, or a creamy cleanser. Rinse your face thoroughly with warm water, followed by cool water to close the pores.

Pat your face dry. Apply a toner (it does not contain alcohol). This toning step is very important because it thoroughly removes all traces of soil. Repeat with fresh pieces of cotton until it comes away from your face clean. If yours is combination skin, concentrate especially on your T-zone.

Now, apply a lightweight moisturizer for normal skin. Do not apply to your oily areas if you have combination skin.

In the evening, cleanse you face with your soap or cleanser. Follow with your toner.

Apply a night cream. It is slightly more concentrated than a daytime moisturizer, sealing in moisture while you sleep. If your skin is combination, avoid the T-zone.

Apply an undereye cream and blot the excess.

DAILY CLEANSING REGIMEN FOR OILY SKIN

Be sure you've given yourself the tissue test and not just assumed you have oily skin. The light's reflection sometimes leaves a glow that may be mistaken for oily skin, when in fact, it is not.

Begin your morning cleansing with a cleanser or soap designed especially for oily skin. Rinse very well, with warm water then with cool water to close the pores.

Pat your face dry. Your next step is to apply an astringent which contains a small amount of diluted alcohol to help remove excess oil and dirt.

Never use plain alcohol. It's too harsh and drying and does nothing to clean the skin.

Apply your astringent with fresh pieces of cotton until it comes away from your face clean. If you live in a warm climate, keep your astringent cool by storing it in the refrigerator. You will find this quite refreshing, too.

Because your skin is already producing a sufficient amount of oil, you do not need to use a moisturizer. Makeups should be water-based. Use powders instead of creams.

You will probably want to refresh your face in the afternoon. You can either cleanse again as you did in the morning, or simply apply first a tissue to blot excess oils, then your cool astringent. Do not overdo use of your astringent, though, because you do not want to irritate your delicate skin.

In the evening, follow the same regimen as in the

morning. Do not apply a night cream, although you may want to apply an undereye cream; blot the excess.

DAILY CLEANSING REGIMEN FOR DRY SKIN

In the morning, begin your cleansing regimen with a creamy cleanser. If you prefer to use soap, it should be designed specifically for dry skin. Rinse with warm water, then with cool water to close the pores.

Lightly pat skin dry, leaving some water to be naturally absorbed into your skin.

Use a mild toning lotion applied with cotton moistened with water (to dilute the toner) to remove remaining soil. Never use a product that contains alcohol. It's too drying for your skin.

Apply the toning lotion with fresh pieces of cotton until it comes away from your face clean.

Use creamy makeups. Avoid powders which may absorb too much of your natural oils.

In the afternoon or whenever you feel the need, lightly spritz your face with purified water. Let the moisture absorb into your skin. You may find it necessary to apply additional moisturizer, too.

In the evening, remove your makeup and cleanse with just a creamy cleanser and moistened cotton. Follow with your toner. Apply a rich emollient night cream liberally, blotting the excess with tissue. Then apply your eye cream, also blotting excess.

The Personalized At-Home Facial

A professional facial is one of beauty's sybaritic experiences. It's your chance to thoroughly clean and nourish your skin while you relax.

A facial provides the complete deep cleansing that goes beyond your daily regimen. It tones and tightens pores to improve your skin's texture. Your circulation is stimulated, which speeds up your skin's elimination of waste materials.

Lydia Sarfati and Shoshana Kliot, skin-care specialists and proprietors of the Klisar Skin Care Center in New York City, have designed this personalized at-home facial for you. Before you begin, here are some basic tips.

DO NOT DISTURB   You should give yourself a facial once every week. Set aside one evening to pamper just you. Designate a room or area where you will not be disturbed, and make it as comfortable as possible.

Take everything you will need with you so you do not risk interruptions. Be sure to wear comfortable clothes or a favorite bathrobe. Keep a blanket handy in case you want to nap during your facial. Take a cold pitcher of water, a glass, and a straw so you can sip while you relax.

Once you firmly establish your beauty routine, your family will understand that this is your time to enjoy the luxury of being a woman!

KLISAR'S RECIPES FOR FACIAL MASKS

Honey-and-Almond Facial Scrub

> 2 teaspoons of uncooked oatmeal
> 1 tablespoon ground almonds
> 1 tablespoon milk
> ½ teaspoon honey

Mix to the consistency of a thick pudding. Apply for ten to fifteen minutes. This mask, recommended for all skin types, tones and nourishes your skin while it deep cleans. You will immediately notice the difference in your complexion.

Yeast Mask for Normal or Combination Skin

Blend yeast with a little water to make a thick paste. Apply for fifteen minutes. This mask has both a tightening as well as a cleansing effect.

Potato Pack for Oily Skin

Peel and grate a raw potato. Using a blunt knife, spread the grated potato to make a thick paste on strips of cheesecloth. Place the strips on forehead, cheeks, and chin, potato side down. Leave the strips on for fifteen to twenty minutes. This paste has a great drawing ability to remove oil and help tighten pores. It also nourishes the skin with vitamins A and B.

Nourishing Mask for Dry Skin

Mix one egg yolk with a heaping tablespoon of honey and the contents of one vitamin E capsule. Apply to face and throat. Leave on for fifteen to twenty minutes. This mask combines the toning qualities of honey with the vitamin B nourishment of egg yolk and the rejuvenating ability of vitamin E.

For Your Facial You Will Need

Eye-makeup remover or mineral oil

Soap or cleanser

Camomile tea

Honey-and-Almond Facial Scrub

Witch hazel

Mask for normal, combination, oily, or dry skin

Toner or astringent

Night cream or moisturizer

Eye cream

Two towels

Nonsterile roll of cotton

Tissues.

Now You Are Ready to

1. Secure your hair away from your face with clips, bobby pins, a hairband, or a mesh hairnet.

2. Remove your eye makeup with the remover pads or with mineral oil. Remove the oil residue with cotton dampened with warm water. Rinse your face with warm water.

3. Massage cleanser into your skin, using upward and outward circular motions. Rinse and repeat, concentrating on your complexion's problem areas. Remove cleanser with cotton that has been saturated with very warm water and repeat until no soil or makeup is left on the cotton.

4. Rinse your face well with warm water.

5. Now you are ready to steam your face. Boil a large pot of water. Remove it from the stove and let it steep with camomile tea for ten minutes. This gives the water time to cool down sufficiently so that it is steaming, but not boiling, hot.

6. Place your pot of herb tea on a table. Sit upright in a chair, with plenty of tissues handy to catch perspiration. Cover your head and the pot with a towel, creating an angle. Do not lean directly over the steaming pot. It can burn your face. Steam for seven to ten minutes. Rinse with warm water, but do not dry your face completely.

7. Next, apply the Honey-and-Almond Facial Scrub to face and neck in upward and outward circular motions. Do not apply to your delicate eye area.

Note: Do not use on acne or irritated skin. You can easily spread infection to the rest of your face.

8. Prepare your eye pads. Mix cool witch hazel (keep the bottle in your refrigerator) with a little bit of water. Dampen two pieces of cotton with cool water and apply the witch hazel/water mixture to the cotton.

9. Relaxation is an important part of your facial. Lie down with your feet elevated to improve circulation. Apply your eye pads to relax your eyes. It takes ten to fifteen minutes to enjoy the complete benefit of your facial scrub.

10. Now, thoroughly rinse your face with warm water, then with cool water to remove all traces of the mask.

11. Next, apply your facial mask for your particular type skin to face and neck, again avoiding your eye area.

12. Using eye pads, rest for fifteen to twenty minutes.

13. Remove the mask completely with cotton dampened with warm water. Then rinse well with warm water, then with cool water.

14. Apply toner or astringent to face and neck. Repeat until cotton comes clean, removing all residue from the mask. This step also tones and tightens pores.

15. Moisturize with eye and night creams if your facial is applied in the evening, or moisturizer, if early in the day.

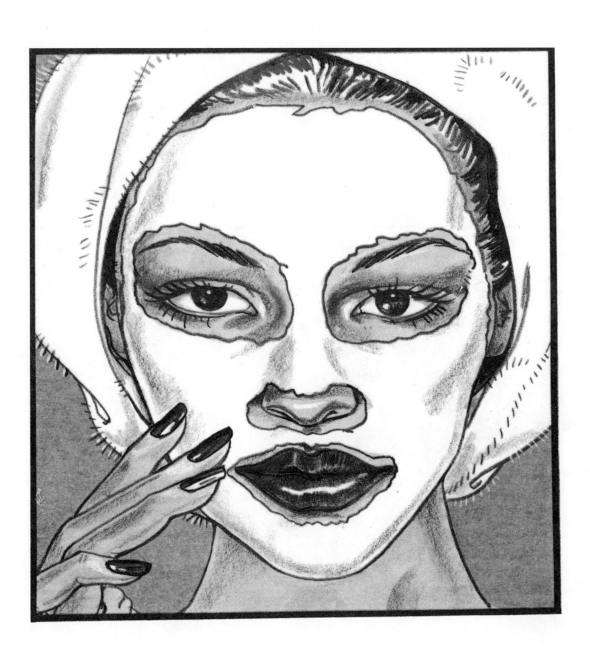

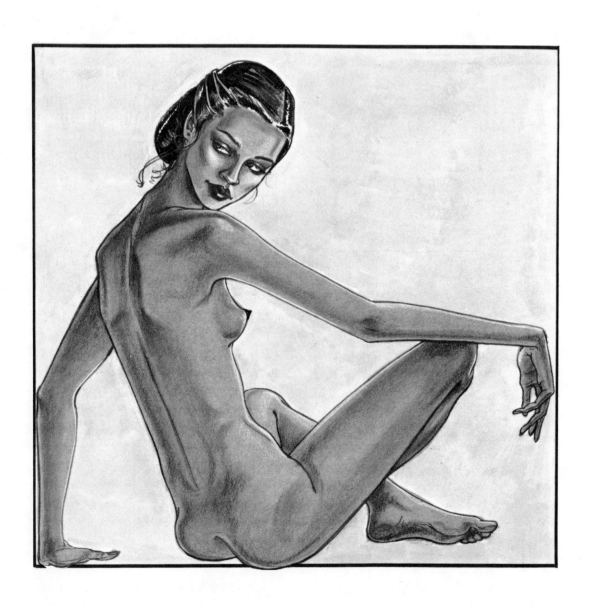

Body Velvet

Your body is the colorful wrapping of the most precious gift you can ever receive—*you*. Keep it velvety smooth, beautiful to look at . . . and to touch.

Make your skin wonderful to be inside of by turning rituals like bath and shower into sensual, pleasurable experiences. Dress your body in layers of fragrance. Do something special for your hands and feet.

SLOUGH YOUR BODY The bath or shower is where you begin to turn your skin into velvet. The body's natural exfoliation process produces a fine layer of dead skin cells. These cells, which are white, leave our skin looking dry and flaky because they form a contrast on dark skins that's not obvious on white skins.

Slough off dead skin cells by epiabrading your body with nature's sponge, the loofah, available in drug and dime stores. The tingly sensation you'll experience is the refreshed feeling of stimulating your body's circulation. Pay special attention to elbows, knees, and the soles of your feet where skin is naturally the roughest.

Since your skin is delicate, take extra care to shop for mild glycerin or superfatted soaps that do not strip skin of natural moisture. In some cases, perfume soaps or soaps with strong ingredients can cause irritations, epecially if your skin is dry and sensitive.

When you cleanse your body, take your time. It responds better to a firm massaging than an abrupt scrubbing.

For special moisturizing, add lots of lubricating bath oil to your tub. Or massage it all over your body *before* you bathe. Don't use soap for your moisturizing bath or you'll remove the extra oil from your skin. Keep soaks warm and short. Long, hot baths can drain your skin of its natural moisture.

Organize your bathroom with the same care and thoughtfulness as you do your kitchen. Are soaps, oils, and bath beads easily accessible? If not, a small investment in a tray for your tub will keep soaps and sponges at arm's reach.

PATTING IN MOISTURE Once you're out of the tub, pat, don't rub, your body with a soft, fluffy towel until it's just moist. Let your skin maximize the benefits of water by absorbing the rest.

It's lack of moisture, not of oils, that leads to dry skin, explains New York dermatologist Dr. George Jordan. In winter when humidity is low, moisture evaporates easily and skin quickly becomes dry and irritated. Because there are more oil glands in the face, back, chest, and upper arms which help to seal in moisture, we notice dryness more on the lower parts of our bodies.

Applying a lightweight moisturizing cream or lotion while the skin is still damp is an effective way to lock in moisture. Liberally massage it all over your body, including tummy and buttocks.

BODY LAYERING Surround yourself with scent by layering with fragrance. You can begin with a scented body lotion, then add the next layer by generously dusting scented powder under arms and all over your body. If you use more than one scent, experiment to make sure they mix well; otherwise, stick to one fragrance.

Add toilet water or cologne, the lightest in the perfume family, to pulse points—behind the ears, at the base of your neck, in the fold of your arms, at the wrist—wherever you feel your pulse beat. Remember that scent rises, so don't forget to dab just below your belly button, ankles, and back of knees, too.

Just before you're ready to leave your home, reinforce your body layering with perfume, the most concentrated form of fragrance. It lasts for hours.

CHOOSING YOUR FRAGRANCE Annette Green, executive director of the Fragrance Foundation in New York, offers the following guidelines to help you choose your fragrance. The oilier your skin the longer your fragrance will last. Dry skins absorbs the scent quicker and require heavier application of fragrances.

Summer heat intensifies the scent of any fragrance which should be lighter than the one worn in winter. Keep a wardrobe of fragrances year round to change your scent with the mood or occasion.

When you shop for fragrance, remember to test before you buy. Your individual body chemistry determines whether or not a particular fragrance is for you.

Sample two fragrances by applying one to each wrist. The *top note* is what you'll smell first. Wait five to ten minutes until the fragrance "settles." When you sniff each wrist again, you'll smell the *middle note.* Now continue shopping and check your wrists in a half hour. The *bottom note,* how the fragrance really smells on you, is the one you should love.

SUMMER SPECIALS Your body needs special attention in summer months or if you live in a warm climate year round. Body hairs, whose function is to trap dust, also trap heat. It's important to keep your body cool by shaving regularly to remove unwanted hair from underarms.

Antiperspirants stop perspiration, but should not be used every day. Eliminating moisture is the natural way to keep the body cool, and you'll perspire heavily in your face if not under your arms.

Alternate with deodorants and dust generously with your scented powder or baby powder which is extra absorbent. Apply, whenever you shower, for added protection.

WAX YOUR BODY Special summer attention is also focused on keeping legs smooth and hair-free. Waxing is one of the best, long-lasting ways to accomplish this, according to Lydia Sarfati. Since waxing effectively removes exfoliated cells, your skin will feel velvety soft, too.

Waxing the bikini area keeps you especially attractive in your swimsuit. Stomach hairs are also easily and painlessly removed. Bikini waxing should only be done by a professional, though, because she can see and reach areas that you cannot. She has the best angle to remove the wax quickly and completely.

If you prefer to shave, use shaving lotion to swell and raise hairs, maximizing the benefits of your razor. Shave first in the direction of hair growth, then in the opposite direction for the closest shave possible. Wait one half hour for pores to close before lathering on body lotion.

POLISHED NAILS   Beautiful hands are the result of good grooming that comes from a weekly manicure. Buffing nails stimulates circulation and polish protects from chipping and splitting.

Your hands deserve pampering. These tips from *Bride's* will help you get the perfect professional manicure so that your nails are always their best.

THE PROFESSIONAL MANICURE

Begin by removing old nail polish with cotton soaked in oily polish remover. Then use the coarse side of an emery board to file nails into smooth oval shapes—not squares or unnatural points. To prevent breakage, file with light strokes in one direction only.

Next, soak fingertips in sudsy water for five minutes. Scrub nails on top and underneath with a soft nail brush. Resoak five minutes. Dry hands and apply cuticle remover to base and sides of nails.

Do not cut cuticles. Instead, gently nudge cuticles back with a cotton-covered orangewood stick. With cuticle clippers, carefully cut hangnails *only*. Wash and moisturize hands.

Using a nail buffer or chamois cloth, buff each nail about thirty times in one direction only. Try a pink-tinted buffing paste to moisturize nails and give them a lustrous, healthy finish. Wash hands to remove excess paste. The smoother surface will help nail polish adhere longer.

Next, use a base coat before polishing, to prevent the polish from staining nails and to guarantee a smooth finish.

Then, from cuticle edge to nail tip, stroke a layer of colored polish just three times—once in the center, once on each side. Allow at least four minutes drying time, then color-coat another sheer layer. To double the life of your manicure, brush a clear sealer over the polish and under nail tips.

After nails dry, dip a cotton swab in remover. Wisk off excess polish from cuticles.

TO PRESERVE YOUR MANICURE

Look at that pretty manicure a lot. It'll discourage nail-chewing, cuticle-biting.

Protect nails and polish from chipping by using a pen or pencil to dial the phone instead of your finger.

Avoid using nail clippers on dry nails. Instead, soak fingertips in warm water for several minutes, then trim softened nails.

Once a month, smooth nail ridges with a mildly abrasive file made especially for nail *tops*.

File calluses off the sides of fingers with the fine side of an emery board.

Cream hands with silky lotion after every washing.

Never shake or stir nail polish. It causes air bubbles. To mix, roll bottle between your hands. To thin polish, drop in remover and reroll.

Patch broken nails with special nail paper and glue kit, or cut all nails to a short length.

If nails are already brittle and cuticles dry, avoid using remover more than once a week. It dries cuticles, makes nails brittle. Buff a little every day to stimulate circulation, and soak nails in warm olive oil to soften cuticles.

Wear lined rubber gloves whenever you wash dishes.

PEDICURE YOUR FEET Feet are always most attractive when pedicured. Follow the same directions as for nails, but add the following steps.

Use a clipper to cut nails straight across, then smooth with an emery board.

Soak feet for ten minutes.

Smooth heels and soles with pumice stone.

Fold tissues lengthwise and weave in and out of toes to separate them before applying polish.

Repeat pedicure every two weeks.

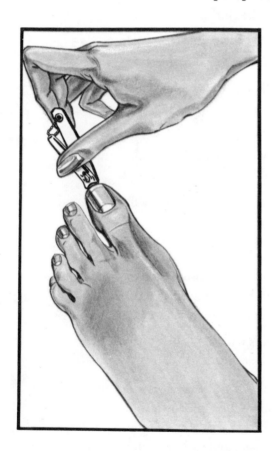

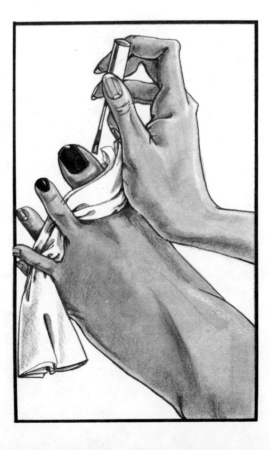

Dr. Muriel Osborne, podiatrist and foot specialist in Washington, D.C., offers this advice to keep your feet healthy.

If your feet are particularly dry, moisturize before and after your bath for special lubrication.

Thick substances coat but do not moisturize your skin. Light creams or lotions that contain lanolin provide maximum benefits.

Be gentle with abrasives, such as pumice stones, on your feet. Remember, they are still skin.

Occasionally, let nails "breathe" free of polish.

Don't sit with legs crossed for long periods of time. This cuts circulation.

Excercise your feet. Point your foot straight, then rotate the ankle in a complete circle, pausing in between to let feet feel the stretch.

Foam-rubber insoles and bicarbonate of soda, or foot powder or spray help check perspiration and odor.

Wear shoes that give complete protection in winter. Open-toe shoes can lead to damage of capillaries and blood vessels from overexposure to the cold.

For daily wear, keep heels no higher than 2½ inches.

Shoes should be immediately comfortable when you try them on. You ruin your feet if you try to "break shoes in" after you buy them.

Buy shoes around three in the afternoon when feet have swelled to their average size.

For serious foot problems, always see a podiatrist.

Sun Savvy

• •

Beaches and vacation spots all over the world are populated with vacationers looking for a healthy, beautiful tan, and that includes Black women and men. Also, sports such as tennis, jogging, swimming, or bicycling encourage active outdoor exercise that exposes us more and more to the wonderful warmth of the sun and are more reasons why we need to understand what our skin is and how best to take care of it.

Getting the right amount of sun supplies essential vitamin D, puts color in your cheeks, and gives you a sense of vitality. But too much sun soaks up moisture, dries and ages the skin. Although black skin requires less protection, we can damage our skin, too, unless we are sun savvy.

IN SEARCH OF A TAN   We know that our skin tans beautifully and easily. Dr. Arthur Sumrall, dermatologist on staff at Winona, Methodist, and St. Vincent's hospitals in Indianapolis, Indiana, explains why.

When exposed to the sun, the skin produces more melanin in an effort to protect it from injury. This color is what we call a "tan." If sun exposure is too much too soon and melanin has not had enough time to form a protective layer to screen out the harmful rays, the skin burns, sometimes becoming raw and blistered.

This constant abuse is one of the major causes of skin cancer. Sun preparations that contain effective ingredients such as PABA (para-aminobenzoic acid), or PABA derivatives, offer the most protection in blocking the penetration of harmful rays beneath the skin's surface.

Black skins need very little additional protection since melanin naturally screens out the sun's harmful rays. But there is a difference between very little protection and none at all, warns Dr. Sumrall. Although skin cancer is rare among Blacks, it can occur. More likely to happen, however, are premature wrinkling and aging of the skin.

FIRST EXPOSURE If you are not used to being out in the sun, the most important time to protect your skin is during your first prolonged exposure. Remember, you can still burn even though you are Black. You may even be sun sensitive to the degree that you get an adverse reaction to too much sun exposure. Or, you may need little or no protection at all.

A Food and Drug Administration advisory panel has set up guidelines for the labeling of products to make it easier for everyone to select the right sun-screen or sun-tan lotion. Products are rated for the amount of sun screen they contain—a low number for minimum sun screen, a high number for maximum protection.

THE SUN-PROTECTION FACTOR Products labeled SPF-2 (Sun-Protection Factor that allows you to stay in the sun twice as long as you could normally) are recommended for dark-complexioned individuals who rarely burn and tan easily. This product offers minimum protection and often contains rich emollients such as coconut oil or cocoa butter.

If you always tan well but do burn occasionally, you need a product marked SPF-4 which offers moderate protection. It allows you to stay in the sun four times longer than you could normally and is recommended for medium skin tones.

SPF-6 is recommended for hard to tan skin—those who usually burn and tan gradually. SPF-8 is for those who always burn and rarely tan. Because this product offers such high protection, it is called a *sun screen* since it prevents sunburn and permits minimal tanning. You can use a sun screen on sensitive areas such as tops of hands or feet, ears, or your husband's bald spot.

If you are sun sensitive, have an allergy to the sun, or don't wish to tan at all, products with the SPF-15 offer maximum protection. They are generally labeled *sun blocks* because they totally block both the tanning and harmful rays of the sun. If you purchase this product in an alcohol base, it may stain white or light-colored clothing, but in the alcohol formulation, it is one of the most effective sun blocks to date.

Dr. Sumrall cautions that baby oil and cocoa butter alone do not contain any sun screen and offer no protection against the rays that can cause aging and skin cancer.

SUN TIPS When sunning, remember to reapply your lotion after every swim, and don't forget tops of ears, hands, and feet. Remember that you can burn right through the water.

When boating, cover up arms and legs very well, both with sun screen and opaque clothing because you're getting twice the amount of rays—that from the sun and what's reflected off the water. A wide-brimmed hat gives additional protection to both face and hair.

When playing in the sun, replenish your body's moisture loss by drinking plenty of water—eight glasses daily.

The sun's rays are strongest from noon to two, and if you're not accustomed to the hot sun, go inside. Don't be misled by a cloudy day. Burning rays are getting through.

Avoid wearing perfume when sunning. Besides attracting insects, ingredients in perfumes may cause allergic reactions when exposed to sunlight and could result in hyperpigmentation.

When you're skiing, remember to wear sun protection, too. The snow reflects just like the water, bouncing those rays right back at you.

Cosmetic Surgery

Society's reward for an attractive appearance, reinforced with every date, interview, or business meeting, is opportunity and success. In addition to being well-educated and informed, the pressure is on for you to look your best in order to gain acceptance and approval. Also, once you look and feel attractive, you can build the necessary confidence and self-esteem to aggressively seek your place in the world.

The woman who is disturbed by her looks (whether it's due to scarring as a result of acne, wrinkled, aged-looking skin, or a nose that's too large for her features) may be shy and less aggressive. Often her deformity is magnified in her mind, and she feels it is magnified in the minds of others, too.

Cosmetic surgery is surgery that improves the appearance. Unlike reconstructive plastic surgery, whose main objective is to restore function and appearance following trauma from accidents or birth defects, cosmetic surgery is corrective surgery to balance facial features or to minimize some of the obvious signs of aging. Cosmetic surgery will not guarantee you fame or success, but it may improve your own self-image so that you may cultivate the innate qualities that allow you to function more confidently.

THE KELOID MYTH The keloid myth is a primary factor that has minimized the availability of cosmetic surgery for Black women. Although operations are readily performed on other parts of her body, doctors often contraindicate cosmetic surgery because of the misconception that because some black skins keloid, all black skins keloid.

What is a *keloid?* According to Dr. Harold E. Pierce, a Philadelphia dermatologist and cosmetic surgeon pioneering in the field of corrective surgery, a keloid is a clawlike lesion or scar that visibly extends beyond the boundaries of a normal scar.

Keloids are commonly confused with *hypertrophic* scars, a scar that has healed incorrectly from a wound or incision.

Keloids form when the scar tissue, instead of normally halting itself, continues to pile up into a large, shiny growth. Melanin, vital in the healing process, encourages the formation of scar tissue, and keloids are more common in dark complexions because of melanin.

Dr. Pierce has had considerable success in the removal of keloids. He accomplishes this by resurfacing the area (removing the keloid) and applying a pressure bandage until the new healing process is complete. The pressure forces the scar to heal flat and prevents it from extending above the surface of the skin. Injections of cortisone and X-ray therapy while the scar reheals enhance the beneficial effects of surgical-scar revision.

A NEW SURFACE Severe cases of acne often leave unsightly scarring, or acne pits, in addition to hyperpigmentation. To date, the most effective method of camouflaging acne scars is through *dermabrasion,* mechanically sanding the skin to create a new, smooth surface.

Because of the keloid myth, dermabrasion, also effective in minimizing hypertrophic scars, is generally precluded for black skins in the majority of cases. Many doctors also fear that hyperpigmentation, which often occurs during the healing process, will leave their patients more dissatisfied than they were with their acne scars.

However, Dr. Pierce has successfully dermabraded black skin for over twenty-five years and feels that, with patience, knowledge, and skill, gratifying results can be equally obtained in black as well as white skins. He explains how.

Dermabrading the entire face produces optimum results. Sharp lines of pigment change can be minimized if the skin is carefully "feathered," especially around the eye area, to avoid an abrupt margin. For the patient with deep acne scars (ice-pick scars), Dr. Pierce recommends two treatments—primary scar revision followed by dermabrasion in six to eight weeks.

Since acne can be physically disfiguring and sometimes mentally disabling, careful re-evaluation of dermabrasion for dark skins must be reconsidered. For the many women affected, a new surface can be a new beginning.

DERMATITIS PAPULOSA NIGRA *Dermatitis papulosa nigra* are tiny black or brown moles which often appear on the face. Doctors do not know the cause, but eight out of ten Black adults develop this condition between the ages of ten and twenty.

The moles are totally benign, and surgical treatment to remove them is purely cosmetic. Dr. Pratibha Arora, assistant professor of Dermatology, Howard University College of Medicine in Washington, D.C., recommends light desiccation and cryotherapy to lift the moles off the skin. He cautions that scraping can produce hyperpigmentation or hypopigmentation.

THE FACE-LIFT *Rhytidoplasty,* or the face-lift, is cosmetic surgery that a growing number of Black women are considering as part of their beauty options. The face-lift tightens sagging skin that makes you look fatigued and older than you feel, and although not inexpensive, it is affordable.

There are two types of rhytidoplasty—full and modified. The latter is a less major procedure that is quite effective if performed before there is excessive wrinkling. It involves removing excess tissue from the cheek and neck area. A full face-lift involves tightening the skin at the temporal area as well. The incision and stitches are hidden in the hairline and behind the ears.

A face-lift does not permanently stop the aging process, but it does give a younger appearance than if you never had the operation. Hospitalization varies from three days to a week, and swelling and discoloration usually subside anywhere from seven days to two weeks.

Fine wrinkles around the lips, eyes, and forehead can be smoothed by a procedure called facial peeling, or *chemabrasion.* Chemicals actually peel away the top layer of skin to reveal fresh, new skin after several weeks. However, since this process involves the use of strong chemicals to remove the surface layer of skin, you may want to discuss the risk of hyperpigmentation with your doctor.

THE EYELIDS You may find that *blepharoplasty*—surgery of the eyelids to remove wrinkles or bagginess caused by hereditary or normal aging—or an operation that flattens the nasolabial fold around your mouth are all the "lifting" your face really needs. These minor procedures are performed more frequently than the full face-lift and produce some of the most dramatic results.

THE EARS   *Otoplasty* is cosmetic surgery to correct deformed, flattened, or protruding ears. It is as equally successful when performed on children as it is on adults. Hospitalization is usually only twenty-four hours.

THE NOSE   *Rhinoplasty* is the name for this procedure that improves the shape and size of the nose so that it is in harmony with other facial features. Excess bone or cartilage is removed and the remainder resculpted. Rhinoplasty produces the same dramatic results as blepharoplasty, but because it involves the restructuring of bones, it can be somewhat painful. It is not until the swelling and discoloration disappear completely and the bandages are removed that you can see the final results. Remember, you cannot select the type of nose you want and expect your surgeon to create a totally new nose for you. He can only work with what you have.

THE LIPS   Oversized lips can also be proportioned to your face through cosmetic surgery. *Cheiloplasty* removes excess tissue from a redundant lower lip so that it is in proportion to the upper lip. In rare instances the upper lip may require surgery, too.

BODY SCULPTING   Cosmetic surgery is not limited to the face and neck. Body sculpting also brings the extremities into proper perspective by removing excess skin and fat from upper arms, abdomen, buttocks, and upper thighs. *Mammaplasty* corrects breasts that may be too large or too small. Deformities of the fingers and toes can be corrected through *orthopedic surgery*.

GREAT EXPECTATIONS   The goal of the cosmetic surgeon is to produce natural features, so often your family and friends may not be immediately aware of any minor changes. The biggest complication with cosmetic surgery is trying to satisfy a woman who has unrealistic expectations, hoping that the end result will make her look like someone else.

Because of the many psychological implications associated with cosmetic surgery, doctors spend an equal amount of time consulting with their patients as they do operating on them. To get a more accurate overview, Dr. Pierce often refers his prospective patients for psychological evaluation before surgery is performed. If he feels the patient really wants a beauty salon, surgery, in these cases, is often denied.

SAME-DAY SERVICE   Some procedures are performed under controlled conditions in the doctor's office, and you can recuperate at home. Even if your operation requires hospitalization, you may return to work in a few days or weeks with your bandages. Realize that it can take several months before the swelling and discoloration subside completely.

Expect restrictions, such as staying out of the sun, along with the discomfort. Follow your doctor's orders to the letter. No operation, no matter how simple it seems to you, is without its risks, and results are never guaranteed. The healing process is as important as the meticulous surgical procedure, and you must co-operate with your doctor for the best results.

KNOW YOUR MEDICAL HISTORY   If you are considering cosmetic surgery, your first task is to review your personal and family medical history. If there has been an incidence of keloidal scarring, you must alert your doctor.

CHOOSING YOUR DOCTOR   Because the success of cosmetic surgery depends upon your doctor's skill, you will want the most qualified surgeon you can find. He must be sensitive to your needs as a Black woman and familiar with your skin so that he can work with you for the best results.

Former patients who are pleased with the results of their surgery are the best testimonials. No reputable surgeon guarantees results, and it's wise to avoid any doctor who makes such promises. The cosmetic surgeon is not a magician. He can only work with what you, the patient, presents. He cannot make you look like someone else. He strives only to make you look *better,* helping you to build your self-esteem by improving your own body image.

Following is a list of some of the most qualified Black cosmetic surgeons who have the interest of you, the Black female, at heart. You can write to them, and if you arrange for a personal consultation, remember that the doctor is granting you his valuable time and may therefore charge you a consultation fee.

Before you make your first appointment, check your doctor's area of specialty—rhinoplasty, dermabrasion, face-lift. If he does not personally perform the procedure you are interested in, he may refer you to another qualified colleague.

René Earles, M.D., 2011 East Seventy-fifth Street, Suite 206, Chicago, Illinois 60649

James W. Hobbs, M.D., 1818 South Western Avenue, Suite 207, Los Angeles, California 90006

Lawrence M. Iregbulem, M.D., FRCS(E), Plastic and Reconstructive Surgeon, Federal Orthopaedic and Plastic Hospital, P.M.B. 1294, Enugu, Nigeria

A. Paul Kelly, M.D., Chief, Division of Dermatology, Martin Luther King, Jr. General Hospital, 12021 South Wilmington Avenue, Los Angeles, California 90059

Harold E. Pierce, M.D., 301 City Line Avenue, Bala Cynwyd, Pennsylvania 19004

Arthur J. Sumrall, M.D., 3231 North Meridan Street, Suite 31, Indianapolis, Indiana 46208

THE PRETTIEST SMILE   Your smile illuminates your face, and beautiful teeth are indicative of good health and careful grooming.

According to New York City dentist Allen M. Bressler, D.D.S., P.C., cosmetic dental surgery corrects the less-than-perfect. In a few visits to your dentist, you can replace missing, chipped, or damaged teeth that can make you feel self-conscious or hesitant to smile. Regular checkups preserve your teeth by catching problems early. (Just as every woman has a general doctor and gynecologist you should have a dentist and see him or her twice a year. Taking the extra daily precautions to thoroughly clean teeth and gums means your breath will be fresh-smelling, too.)

Your teeth are a valuable lifetime investment. You will be rewarded each time you look into a mirror or are complimented on your beautiful teeth—and smile!

Makeup

The Optical Illusion

Makeup artistry is skill in creating the perfect optical illusion. Use of light and dark colors accents cheekbones. Warm face tones add subtle highlights to hair and skin. Molding the eyes with smoky colors adds mysterious depth. Defining lips with sheer, soft touches creates wet sensuality . . . all to polish a more beautiful you.

The information in this section helps you master this art by first selecting the right beauty tools and organizing your makeup wardrobe so it is accessible and portable. Understanding how to select colors to best complement your individual skin tone minimizes some of the "error" in trial and error when you shop for cosmetics.

You will also learn a few simple tricks for contouring and highlighting from the professional who fashions the Broadway stars. Step-by-step color makeovers illustrate how easy it is to be your own makeup artist. And for special-occasion makeup, a dancer turned makeup artist offers his unique tips.

With our kaleidoscope of colors, Black women enjoy the widest range of makeup shades. Knowing how to apply your makeup with skill means you are always putting your best face forward.

Getting Organized

• — • — • — • — • — • — • — • — • — • — • — • — • — • — • —

The most important step in your makeup application is having all items and tools neatly organized. There is a trick to this, of course, and who knows better than makeup artists who fashion top models for your favorite magazines.

They must keep their cosmetics compact and easy to carry to photography sittings. Their storing "secret" is inexpensive and is the perfect solution for keeping your makeup handy around your home.

TACKLING YOUR MAKEUP   A plastic fishing-tackle box, approximately six inches wide and twelve inches long, is ideal for storing makeup. The folding trays have different-sized compartments where you can store lipsticks, pots of gloss, and mascara. The bottom of the box has extra room for larger items like compacts and foundations.

Plastic tackle boxes come in several pretty colors and are easy to clean. For that long vacation, you'll find it light enough to carry along with you on the plane. You can purchase one from your hardware, dime, or department store.

PERFECT PORTABLES   For carrying items in your handbag, a small, plastic-lined makeup case conveniently holds everything you need. In case of spills, the plastic will protect both your makeup case and your handbag.

Before you begin your makeup application, you will need these tools of the trade:

Sponges. Great for applying your foundation base. Small natural sponges work best. Always dampen sponge before applying foundation, and wash after each use.

Tweezers. Flat-tip or automatic tweezers are easiest to use.

Eyelash Curler. To curl lashes before applying mascara. Always check to make certain the tiny rubber cushion is in place before using the curler. Without it, you can clip your lashes in half.

Eyebrow Brush and Comb. Keeps your eyebrows neat and separates lashes after applying mascara.

Eyebrow Pencil. Light, medium, dark brown or black, depending on your coloring.

Lip-liner Pencil. A shade darker than your lipstick. A complete wardrobe of pencils is inexpensive and fun to have. If they get too soft to sharpen, store them in your refrigerator for a few hours.

Lipbrush. The best way to apply your lipstick unless yours already has a sponge-tip applicator.

Powder Brush. Very fat, soft, rounded tips make dusting your face easy.

Contour Brush. Flat at the tip. The bristles are held firmly together to shade temples, cheeks, chin, nose.

Cotton Swabs.

Cotton.

Tissues.

Keep all beauty tools—brushes, sponges, combs—clean by sudsing them with mild soap and very warm water. Always apply makeup with clean items.

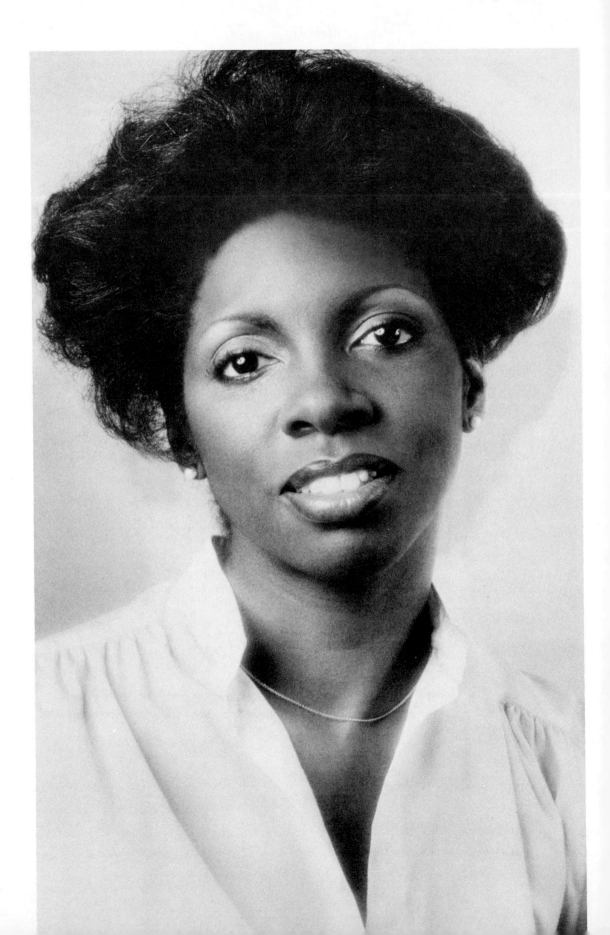

Texture on Texture

Complementing natural skin tones by coloring with makeup is adding texture on texture. Your complexion, with its own vibrancy, warmth, and richness, comes really alive when highlighted with just the right touch of color.

Your skin color *is* your first cosmetic, your initial texture. Each makeup shade you add is like layering a sweater or scarf over a blouse, adding more texture to create the perfect harmony.

Some shades play up your natural complexion more than others. How do you choose from the multicolored palette of makeup colors? Here are a few basic tips that are not hard-and-fast rules, but general guidelines to help you in your makeup selection.

UNDERSTAND UNDERTONES Black women have a wide variety of *undertones*—yellow, orange, red. This color you see in *addition* to your pigment is your guideline to selecting your complete range of makeups, from foundation to eye shadows. Each color will blend or contrast, depending on your undertone.

MATCHING THE FOUNDATION The purpose of your foundation is to make your complexion even, in order to establish a uniform base for your makeup. Your foundation should be the same color as your skin.

This presents a challenge for us because it is impossible for cosmetic companies to produce a makeup base for each hue gradation in Black women. There is, however, a common denominator.

When you select your foundation base, choose a color that matches your undertone. In addition to the depth of the brown foundation color, also select the base for its golden quality if your undertone is yellow, copper quality if yours is orange, or rose if yours is red.

If you have a mixture of undertones, select your base from your deepest undertone. Even if the foundation is slightly lighter or darker than your skin, it will blend well because the basic tones between your skin and the makeup are the same.

CONTRASTING WITH BLUSH   Your blush color adds a healthy glow to your complexion. It complements your makeup and frames your face by emphasizing your cheeks, jaw, and brow areas. The blusher shade you choose should offer subtle contrast to your natural undertones.

For example, a rose tone can be a beautiful highlighter for yellow undertones. Intensify the depth of your blush color with the depth of your skin color. Choose a soft rose if you are fair complexioned, more intense rose if you are browner.

Coral complements orangey undertones, and a pale coral blush for lighter complexions accents as beautifully as deep corals for darker complexions. Vivid pink and plums give a natural glow to reddish undertones.

CHANGING COLORS   When you purchase eye makeups, remember that the actual color will change on your eyes when combined with your undertones.

If your undertone is yellow, for instance, and you choose a navy blue eye shadow, the color is going to vary slightly when applied to your skin. The lighter your complexion, the truer the color will be. If you are browner, your color will have a more muted quality.

If you wear glasses, your lenses magnify your eye makeup. Remember to keep your colors soft.

Your Facial Map

Once you "map" and analyze the individual structure of your face, you can choose the makeup techniques that are best for you. All it takes is a little concentration to learn how to tweeze your eyebrows, contour and highlight your eyes, nose, cheeks, and lips.

To begin, make yourself comfortable in front of a mirror. You should not have on any makeup. Pull your hair back so you can see all of your face. Have a ruler, pencil or orange-wood stick for easy measuring. Now, follow these basic tips from makeup artist Stanley James.

THE FRAME Your eyebrows are the frame for your face. When you tweeze, you want to create a curved arch that lifts and opens your eyes. Always pluck in the same direction as the hair grows.

Brush your brows up so you can see what their actual line is. Begin by tweezing underneath from the inside bushy edge to the outer edge of your brow. Do not tweeze so that you have an inverted V or a straight line. You want to create a natural, curved arch with the high point two-thirds past the inside corner of the eye.

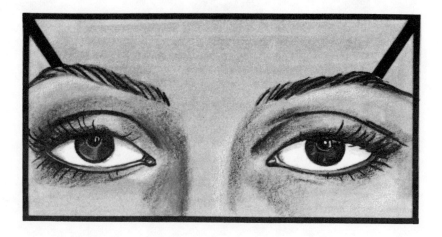

Your eyebrows should begin and end on the same level. If your brows are shaped so that they go all the way up at the ends, you will always look "surprised."

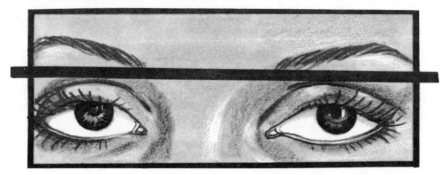

The outside edge should feather to a halt and not extend beyond the angle from your nose to the corner of your eye. If your eyebrows are naturally short, fill in the edge with an eyebrow pencil. Make tiny, short strokes instead of a long, thin line.

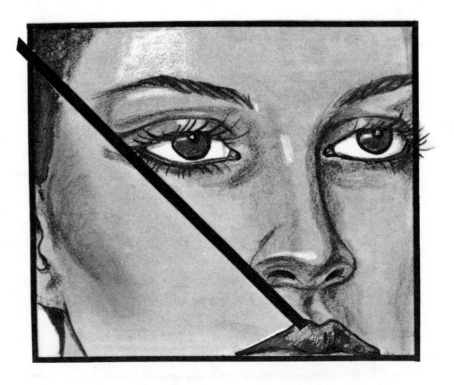

To tweeze stray hairs between your brows, measure from your nose to the inside corner of your eye. You may have to tweeze on top of your brows to remove stray hairs but never to reshape them.

After you tweeze, apply a bit of witch hazel or skin toner to cotton and place this on your brow for a few seconds. This sterilizes the area and helps reduce swelling.

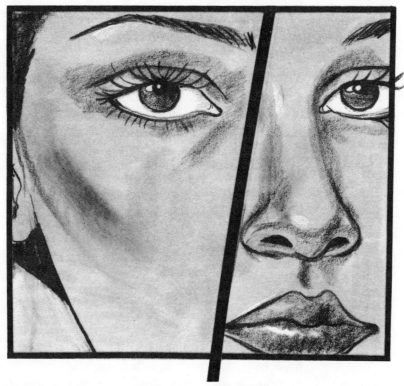

CONTOURING AND HIGHLIGHTING Contouring and highlighting bring out the best points of your facial structure by accentuating bones you may not even be aware of. Wherever you contour, you highlight because one makes the other happen.

The contour color is a dark color, usually three shades deeper than your foundation base. It makes whatever area it is applied to recede or look smaller.

Around every contour use a highlight, a color three shades lighter than your foundation. The highlight makes an area protrude or look larger. It can be an undereye cover or a lighter foundation base.

With contouring and highlighting, the most important step is to blend the colors very well with your sponge or fingertips. They should float into each other at the edges without any sharp lines of demarcation.

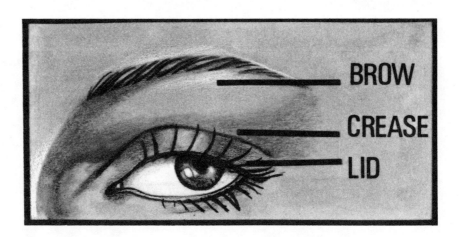

THE FOCAL POINT   Your eyes are the focal point of your face and your makeup gives them depth so that they appear larger, bigger.

There are three areas for eye makeup—the brow bone, crease, and lid. Your *brow bone* is where you apply the highlight colors like pink, salmon, beige, or dusty rose. To find your brow bone, feel with your fingertips.

Your *crease* is the center part and is the area directly beneath the brow bone. This is where you apply your contour colors like plum, burgundy, brown, navy blue, black.

Your crease continues from right under your brow bone to the top of your *eyelid,* the tiny strip of flesh where your lashes are. The color you apply here complements your iris. Generally, avoid using baby blue or bright greens. They are too overpowering on dark skins.

You can make your eyes appear closer together or farther apart by contouring and highlighting. First, know whether they are wide-set or close-set.

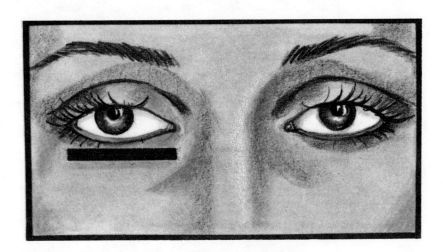

MEASURING YOUR EYES   The distance between your eyes should be equal to the width of one eye. If your eyes are less than the width of one eye apart, they are close-set. If they measure wider than one eye, they are wide-set.

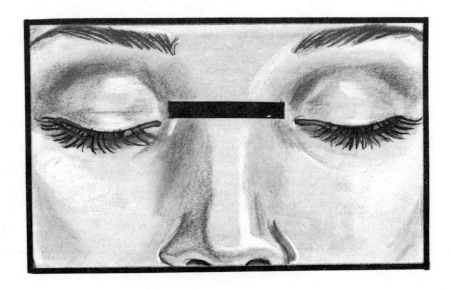

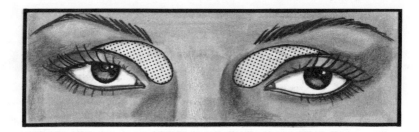

To bring *wide-set* eyes closer, contour on the inside of the crease, near the bridge of your nose, and highlight on the outside.

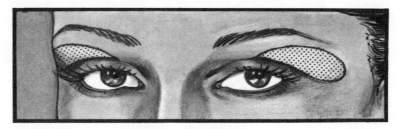

If your eyes are *close-set,* contour on the outside of your crease and highlight on the inside.

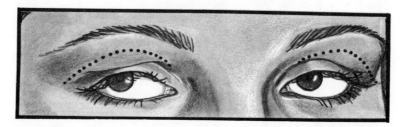

If your eyes are *evenly spaced*, begin your contour on the inside of the crease and extend it to the outside.

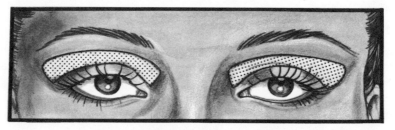

To correct very *fleshy* eyes, use a contour on the folding area to camouflage it, blending right up toward your brow bone. Softly highlight the brow bone.

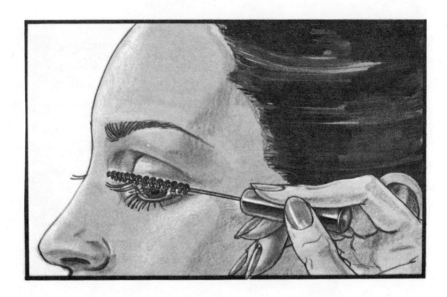

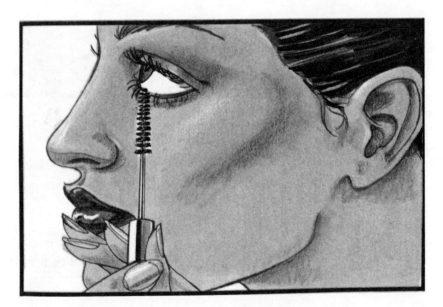

EYE ACCENTS Mascare accentuates your lashes, making them look long
and full. The result—eyes that look dramatically big.

Applying your mascara involves four simple steps: First,
curl lashes. Then, roll the mascara wand over the top of your
lashes. Then roll underneath. Let this dry while you brush the
tip of your wand across your bottom lashes. Repeat for a second
coat. Separate lashes with your lash comb.

SHAPING YOUR NOSE Contouring and highlighting sculpts your nose for a well-defined shape. If you do not have a contour powder, eye shadow works just as nicely. Use your crease color—plums or browns, but not black or navy. They'll make your face look "dirty."

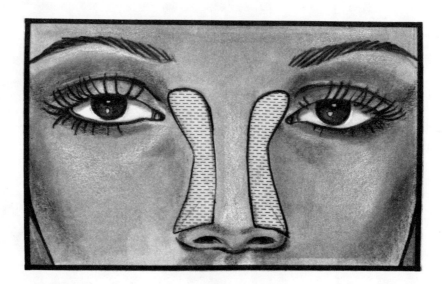

Apply contour with the rubber-tipped applicator that comes with powder eye shadows. This gives a thin, even line. Begin from the corner of your eye along the sides of your nose and blend to a faint line just above the nostrils.

For a soft, natural highlight, apply your undereye cover lightly along the center of your nose. Blend well with your fingertips.

If you want to *shorten* your nose, highlight with a light-colored cream, powder, or foundation. Apply it from the bridge to where your nostrils begin. Blend so there is just a hint of color.

To *lengthen* your nose, begin your highlight at your brow level. Blend to the very tip of your nostrils.

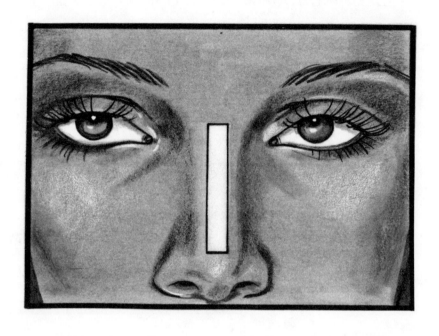

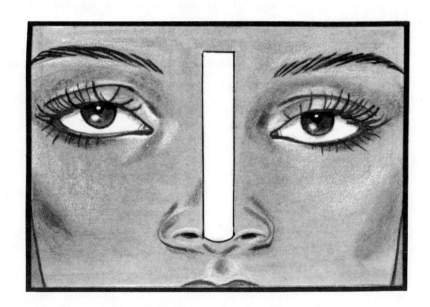

DEFINING YOUR MOUTH   Outlining your mouth is based on the same principle as contouring and highlighting. The darker color on the outside shapes and defines, while your lip color becomes your highlight.

Using a pencil a few shades deeper than your lipstick color, draw along the edge of your lips. Apply lip color with your lipbrush and blot to softly smudge the outline and the color together.

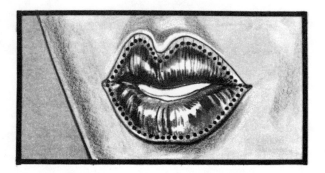

If your mouth is full, outline slightly inside your lips as the dots illustrate in the diagram above, then fill in with two lip colors. The darker color goes right next to your outline; the lighter color fills in the rest.

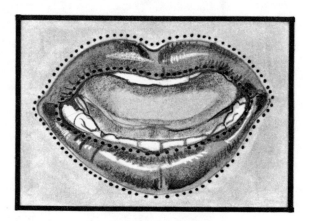

If your mouth is thin, outline at the very edge of your lips. Do not draw outside because this looks artificial. Fill in with your lip color, then open your mouth to color completely inside your lips.

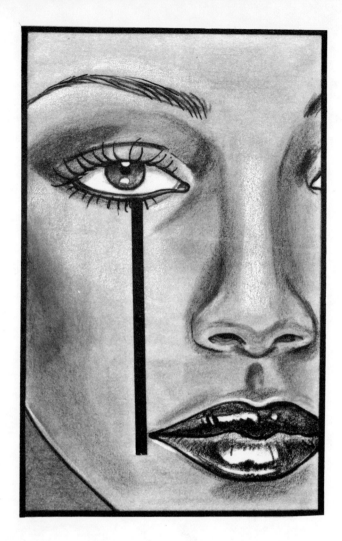

If your mouth extends beyond the center of your eye, it is wide. When you outline, end the line before you reach the corners of your mouth. Fill in with your lip color inside the line.

If you have combinations such as a thin, wide mouth, vary these general rules accordingly.

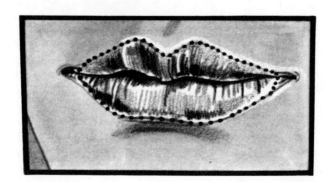

EMPHASIZING CHEEKS Prominent cheekbones mold your face. To emphasize them, contour underneath the bone, in the hollow of your cheek. To find it, feel with your finger. This space below the cheekbone is where you apply your contour with the flat-tipped contour brush. Be sure to blend edges well.

Now, feel again, placing your fingertips right on the cheekbone. See how it continues into your hairline? Apply your blusher here, on top of the bone. Your blush serves as a highlight and the edges should feather into the contour color.

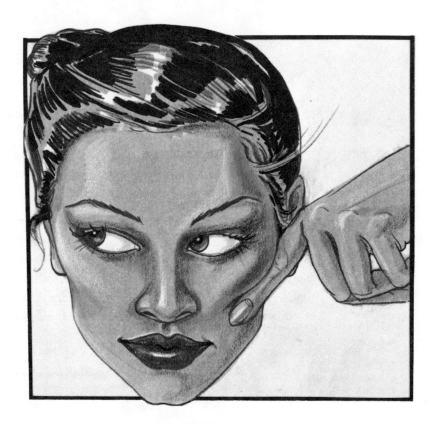

Step-By-Step Real-People Makeovers

• - • - • - • - • - • - • - • - • - • - • - • - • - • - • - • - • - • - •

Makeup is fun! With a little know-how, you can transform yourself into a glamorous, stunning beauty.

These step-by-step real-people makeovers show you everything you need to know to make the most of your natural good looks. Stanley, who designed the hair and makeup for *The Wiz, Timbuktu, Bubbling Brown Sugar,* and *Raisin,* brings his very special hair and makeup expertise to each of the women in these seven pages. Step-by-step photographs in the color section illustrate just how easy applying makeup can be.

You can duplicate techniques from one makeover or combine steps from each. Whether you're a mother, career woman, student, or mature woman, there's beauty information here, just for *you.*

ESTHER—Young Mother/Psychiatric Social Worker   Esther Downing has a beautiful golden-bronze complexion. She is blessed with flawless skin which is normal to dry. Her oval-shaped face allows her lots of versatility when she styles her hair.

We used Esther to illustrate seven basic steps to the perfect daytime makeup. Later, Stanley intensified her makeup, transforming Esther into a ravishing nighttime beauty.

Step 1

Stanley began Esther's makeup application with undereye cover three shades lighter than the foundation to minimize the dark area under her eyes. A light foundation base works just as well as an undereye cream. Stanley patted inward to avoid pulling the delicate skin around her eyes.

(Undereye cover can also be used to hide dark spots of hyperpigmentation. Pat, don't rub, the cover-up right onto the spot you want to conceal. Let this set before applying foundation.)

Step 2

The dots on Esther's temple are her foundation base that matches her yellow undertones. To get the most even coverage, Stanley blended the foundation downward, onto eyelids, lips, feathering into her hairline and neck for a smooth matte finish. Blending upward as if the foundation were a moisturizer gets the foundation into the pores resulting in "spotty" coverage.

To seal the base, Stanley lightly dusted with translucent powder. Now that the "canvas" was set, Esther was ready for color.

Step 3

Using a bright turquoise pencil, Stanley lined Esther's lid and crease area. He blended with a cotton swab until there was only a soft, feathery smudge. To really open her eyes, he angled up at the outer corners.

Stanley dotted undereye cover on Esther's brow bone, too, doubling it as a highlighter.

Step 4

Two coats of black mascara over and under lashes and brows brushed up really opened Esther's eyes.

Step 5

The wine-colored dots are where Stanley applied Esther's blush. He smoothed the blush right onto Esther's cheekbone, into her hairline. To add a warm glow to her face, he blushed the tip of her chin, center brow, sides of temple. Because Esther has such well-defined cheekbones, she didn't need any contouring for her daytime makeup.

Step 6

Stanley outlined Esther's lips with a brown lip-lining pencil. He carefully drew an even line to emphasize the shape of her mouth.

Step 7

Stanley filled in Esther's lip color with a wine red that matched her blush. He used a lipbrush to color right over the foundation. He softened the outline with a cotton swab and blotted for subtle color.

HAIR An off-the-center part and full, fluffy rather than tailored, sleek styles bring the attention right to where it belongs—to Esther's cheeks and eyes.

FROM DAY TO NIGHT To change Esther's looks for evening without changing her daytime makeup Stanley smudged a dark brown liner to the outer corners of her eyes. For drama, he added a smoke burgundy contour to her cheeks. Lip color was intensified and topped with plum gloss. For a shimmery highlight, he dusted gold-flecked powder to brow, cheeks, and collarbone.

Her hair was swooped up in the back, with soft, wispy tendrils framing her face.

Esther—glamorous by day, dazzling at night!

SYLVIA—College Student   Sylvia Davis has a soft, caramel complexion with orange undertones. Her young skin is very oily. Sylvia's hair is candy-cotton soft and she wears it natural, controlling the thickness by pulling it back into a bun.

MOISTURIZING CONDITIONER   Stanley began Sylvia's makeover with a shampoo and moisturizing conditioner. For the conditioner, he mixed three parts castor oil, one part olive oil, and one-half part mineral oil and massaged this into her scalp and hair.

With a hot, damp towel wrapped around her head which was then covered with a shower cap, Sylvia sat under the dryer for twenty minutes to maximize the effects of her deep, penetrating treatment. Afterward, Stanley shampooed again to remove every trace of the oil.

A MINIFACIAL   Now, Stanley turned his attention to Sylvia's skin. He applied a deep-cleansing mask to absorb oils and lift surface impurities. Sylvia relaxed for twenty minutes, then her face was first rinsed with warm water followed by a cool-water rinse to close her pores.

Afterward, Stanley applied an astringent to remove all traces of the mask and to tone the skin. Sylvia's skin looked fresher, clearer, brighter.

A SHORT CUT   Stanley felt Sylvia's long hair made it difficult to work with its natural texture. To make it more manageable, he cut and shaped her hair.

While her hair was still wet, Stanley cornrowed it and set the ends on large permanent rods, using end papers. This gave the ends a curl and kept them from frizzing. Sylvia sat under the dryer for about forty-five minutes.

SOFT MAKEUP   Once her hair was dry, Stanley applied the makeup while the cornrows cooled. He wanted to keep her colors soft and light, appropriate for a young, college-age woman.

For a foundation base, Stanley used pancake makeup applied with a damp sponge. The powder in the pancake makeup absorbs excess oils from overactive, oily skin and helps makeup last longer, too.

Stanley contoured Sylvia's eyes with a coffee color eye shadow blended at the outer half of the lid and in the crease. He brushed a salmon-color shadow over her lids and used this same color as a brow highlighter.

To define her eyes, Stanley smudged a dark brown pencil along the bottom rim and used this same pencil to fill in the edges of her eyebrows.

Stanley curled Sylvia's lashes with an eyelash curler, then applied two coats of black mascara to make her lashes look their longest.

Her cheek color, a deep salmon, was brushed on chin and temples, too. Stanley outlined the lips with a burgundy pencil and filled in lightly with a soft frosted-pink lip color. Gloss blended the two colors together.

PRETTY NATURALLY   Now Sylvia was ready for the final touch. Stanley loosened the cornrows and fluffed her hair. To add even more texture to her soft hair, Stanley randomly twisted the ends to create a frizzed halo.

Sylvia was complete. She looked youthful, radiant, genuinely beautiful.

ARLENE—*Account Supervisor with teenage daughter* Arlene Fridie's clear complexion is a mellow bronze. She has hushed red undertones. Her face is full and round. Arlene likes the variety of changing her hair with her moods and her makeover involves three dramatic new looks.

SHEER MAKEUP To play up Arlene's supple, glowing skin, Stanley applied only the sheerest of foundation to even her complexion. A light dusting of translucent powder allowed her natural coloring to really come through.

Since Arlene's face is full, her small eyes needed to look as big and wide as possible. Stanley chose a beige eye shadow and applied it right up to her brow bone. He contoured only at the outer edges, blending with a smoky-mauve eye shadow. Lining the eyes makes them look smaller, so Stanley did not rim with a pencil. Instead, he applied lots of mascara for thick lashes.

To highlight Arlene's undertones, Stanley used a raspberry blush highlighted over cheeks, temples, and chin. Lips were outlined with a burgundy pencil, smudged with sheer raspberry lip color.

IT'S A WIG! Wig designer André Douglas chose three of his favorite wigs to illustrate the new wig fibers that resemble Black hair so closely not even your hairdresser can tell "it's a wig!"

SPORTY Arlene's sporty look is with "Brownie," a short, curly style she can even swim in.

PARTY For letting her hair down, Arlene prefers something just a bit different. "Nona" is a wash-and-wear look that can be worn as is or twisted and rolled.

SOPHISTICATE For an elegant evening, Arlene looks fabulous in this loose, curly wig. "Miss M" has natural bounce and body, just like her own hair.

MADELINE—Mature Woman Madeline Cleare is a naturally attractive woman whose rich chocolate complexion has subtle yellow undertones. To keep her lovely gray hair luminous, she uses a rinse to make its color come alive. Regular salon visits keep her défrisage soft, pretty, and natural-looking.

MAXIMIZING YOUR LOOKS Madeline's makeover illustrates how any mature woman can maximize her good looks. Makeup that is contemporary and up-to-date demonstrates that, like good wine, a woman has aged well.

BEFORE Madeline takes care of her skin, and this is apparent in its clear, smooth texture. Even without makeup, she is a striking woman.

COVER-UP Stanley began Madeline's makeup with a deep tan undereye concealer to cover up her circles. He also applied the cover-up to the dark crease in her smile line to help it fade away.

    To blend the cover-up, he patted with the fleshy part of his fingertips, feathering the edges.

FOUNDATION Using a damp cosmetic sponge, Stanley blended the foundation base downward with a color that matched Madeline's chocolate complexion exactly. He covered her eyelids and lips, too, blending the foundation right into Madeline's hairline.

POWDER To set the foundation, Stanley dusted with translucent powder (including eyes and lips). The fat powder brush guarantees light, even coverage.

EYE SHADOW Madeline's eyes are naturally deep set, so Stanley did not have to contour. He wanted the colors to be soft and neutral, complementary to both her skin and hair color. The more mature a woman, the softer her eye makeup should be, so Stanley blended two shadows together: plum and navy. He applied this with a sponge-tip applicator in tiny strokes until he covered her entire lids.

    Stanley highlighted the brow bone with undereye concealer to emphasize Madeline's deep-set eyes. He placed a dot at the highest point of the brow bone and blended it outward and up-ward into the eyebrow.

LINER   Heavy, painted lines give a dated, old-fashioned look. Instead, Stanley selected a medium-blue pencil to underline Madeline's eyes. Blue rimmed around the eyes makes the whites of the eyes look whiter and is much softer for mature women than a black pencil. Light-complexioned women should use a lighter blue or comparable color—never too dark.

Stanley began the line at the middle of the bottom rim and continued to the outer corner. He smudged with a cotton swab until there was only a hint of a line left.

EYEBROWS   Using an eyebrow brush, Stanley brushed Madeline's brows up, then filled in for an even line with tiny strokes of a dark brown eyebrow pencil.

Two coats of black mascara completed her eye makeup.

LIP LINE   Makeup for the mature woman should be kept subtle, so Stanley lined Madeline's lips with a maroon rather than a dark brown pencil. He defined her lips by lining along the outer edges of her mouth. Lining the lips also prevents lip color from seeping into any tiny, fine lines around the mouth.

BLUSH   Stanley selected a deep burgundy color for Madeline's cheeks. He brushed it right on her cheekbone, into her hairline, in light, sweeping strokes.

LIP COLOR   A red-raisin color, filled in with a lipbrush for even application, polished Madeline's lips. Stanley blotted with tissue to remove excess color.

AFTER   With Madeline's makeup complete, Stanley fluffed her hair higher at the crown area to balance her square face.

Madeline, who never used to wear makeup, was transformed into a breathtaking beauty. Looking great is part of what getting older is all about. Isn't it?

Image

Completing Your Beautyscope

• •

The care with which you nourish your body, style your hair, cleanse you skin, and apply your makeup indicates how you feel about yourself. It is your total beauty personality, or what I call your *beautyscope*.

Being in touch with your beautyscope involves understanding and loving who you are. Your aim is to improve your looks, not to become someone else. Confidence, and the ability to express it through everything you do, is the signature of feeling and looking great.

The preceding chapters have supplied you with all the basics. Here, in this section, is a little spice to add extra flair to your beauty personality. You'll find tips for special occasions, including sophisticated makeup techniques from a real pro, how to analyze your body from a leading fashion magazine editor, and how to organize and shop economically from a noted fashion and beauty consultant.

When you blend your individual taste, add a dash of character and season it with the knowledge shared by all the specialists in this book, you have all the ingredients to realize the treasures of your own true beauty. Now, *you* are the expert!

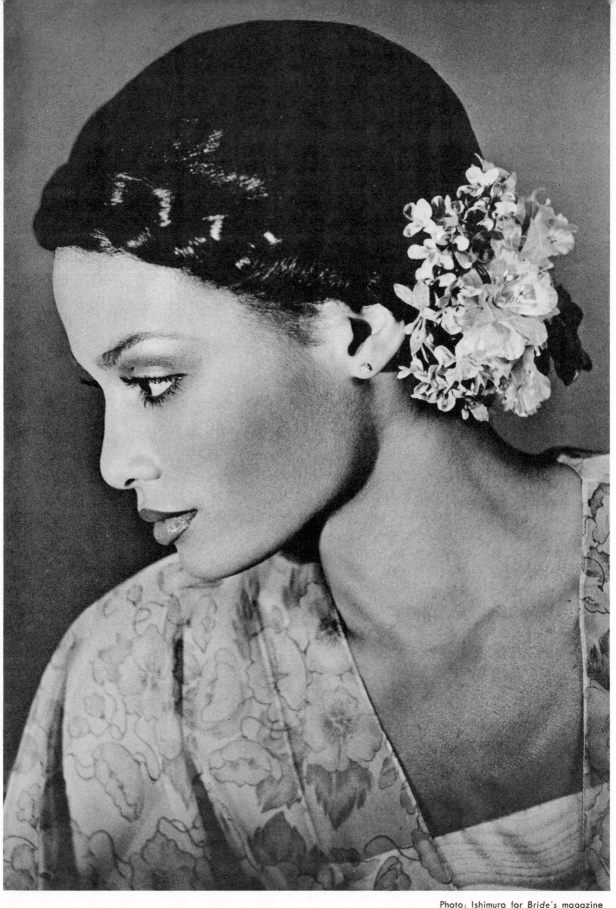

Photo: Ishimuro for *Bride's* magazine
Makeup: Vincent Nasso
Hair: Raul Barbieri

Special Tips for Special Occasions

• •

Events that are monuments in your personal history—weddings, proms, dinner parties—are special occasions when you want to remember yourself, and be remembered, as looking absolutely gorgeous. During the affair you can relax, with the assurance that your hair and makeup are perfect.

Humidity, nervousness, perspiration—all contribute to making you unraveled, especially, it seems, at those times when you want to look and feel your best. How can you relax so you can get to sleep the night before? Is there a check for nervous perspiration? How can you rainproof your hair, have makeup that will last all day?

The special tips in this chapter will help you find the answers so that whatever your special occasion, you can look as great as you feel!

CHANNELING ADRENALINE Feeling excitement is wonderful. It's the happy anticipation of a moment long waited for. Your adrenaline flows, your heart and mind race, and the result is a complete bundle of nerves.

Your first challenge is to calm down by channeling your energies constructively. Exercise is the best way to help combat nerves. It gives your body a specific vehicle for releasing tension. And since your mind has to concentrate on jumping rope, for instance, it's difficult to do so and worry about something else at the same time.

If your exercises are aerobic, do them several hours before your bedtime. Strenuous exercise at night wakes up your body and it may be difficult for you to fall asleep. Yoga exercises are wonderful muscle relaxers and are good for helping you calm down—anytime.

RENEWING THE BODY   Sleep helps the cell-renewal process that keeps your skin looking fresh. It's the most effective method of revitalizing your body.

Missing a night of sleep because of tension or nervous excitement robs your skin and body of the vital energy they need to keep you glowing. These tension-relaxing exercises borrowed from yoga will help you release tension so you can fall asleep easily and soundly.

RELAXING FOR SLEEP

Lie flat on your back with feet apart and arms slightly away from your body. Beginning with your left leg, raise it a few inches off the bed and stretch it, tensing it as tightly as you can. Count slowly to five, tensing tighter and tighter.

Now, release your leg, letting it drop quickly. Roll it from side to side. It is relaxed. Don't think about it anymore.

Repeat the same procedure with your right leg.

Raise your left arm several inches off the bed. Stretch your arm while clenching your fist into the tightest ball you can make. Count to five, clenching tighter and tighter.

Now drop it, roll it from side to side, and forget about it.

Bring your attention to your buttocks. Squeeze them together so tightly that you are slightly elevated off the bed. Do not move any other part of your body. Concentrate on squeezing tighter and tighter until you count to five. Release.

It's time to relax your abdomen. Open your mouth wide and inhale as much air as you can until your stomach is totally expanded. Keep pushing for a slow count of five. Release quickly so that all the air just gushes out of your mouth.

Close your mouth and inhale deeply through your nose, filling up your entire chest. Hold, then open your mouth and let the air rush out.

Raise your shoulders and, without moving your arms, press them together, tightening as much as you can. Hold; release.

Open your mouth wide and stretch your tongue from inside your throat. At the same time, open your eyes as wide as they can go, pushing your eyebrows upward toward the head of the bed. Your entire face should feel the pull and stretch. Count; relax.

Next, squeeze your face into a tiny little ball. Squeeze eyebrows, eyes, mouth, cheeks, neck, all toward a tiny imaginary dot on your nose. Your face will feel like a prune; squeeze it tighter and tighter, then relax.

Now that every muscle has been tensed and relaxed, without moving, take a mental trip to each area of your body. Begin with your left leg. Let your mind make certain all muscles are quiet and relaxed. If an area is tense, let your mind relax it, but don't move. Continue your mental trip in the exact steps as you did to tense and relax.

Before you are completed, you should drift off to a restful night of sleep. . . .

CHECKING PERSPIRATION Perspiration can be embarrassing and annoying, especially on an important day. There's really no way you can stop perspiring altogether, but you can decrease it and check odor.

Remove hair from underarms two or three days before your special day. You can even have them waxed professionally. If you prefer to shave, you may want to repeat it the morning of your big day.

The night before, take a warm relaxing bath (remember, not too long) or shower. Apply your antiperspirant before you go to bed so it can work while you sleep. In the morning, apply your deodorant. Do not use antiperspirants every day because they interfere with your body's normal cooling function.

Dust generously with baby powder. Let this set, and dust again. If you tend to perspire heavily, wear dress shields to protect your clothing.

NAIL WRAPPING   Nothing can ruin your manicure as much as one short, broken nail. Wrap it back together with any of the nail-mending kits available in drug or dime stores.

You can also have your nails artificially extended through nail sculpting. An acrylic substance actually adheres to your own nail with a special glue. You can file, shape, and polish as if the nails were your own. Nail-sculpting kits can be purchased at drug or dime stores, or you can have it done professionally. One word of caution: It's important for your own nails to breathe, so sculpt your nails only when absolutely necessary.

For chip-proof nail polish, manicure the day before, following directions on page 126. The morning of your event, add three more sheer coats of polish—two of color and one top sealer.

ALL-DAY MAKEUP   Makeup artist Bruce Hawkins offers his special tips for the prettiest makeup guaranteed to last all day—and night!

Before you apply foundation, apply your highlighter—a cover cream three shades lighter than your foundation—to tops of cheekbones, chin, nose, and to the middle of your forehead, in addition to under your eyes.

When your foundation is applied over this, it is automatically "lifted" one color in these areas, revealing dark and light shadows on your face, contouring your bones.

After you've applied the foundation, lighten under your eyes again with your cover cream. Also highlight above your lips and around your jawline to add even more contrast when you apply the rest of your makeup.

Now, dust your face with powder. For a smooth finish, mix your translucent powder with a small amount of baby powder. It absorbs moisture and will keep your natural oils from seeping through your makeup so that it will last. The baby powder takes on the natural color of your skin once it "sets."

Lightly dampen your face with a clean, moist cosmetic sponge. You have now "sealed" your base and are ready for color.

GLITTERING EYES   To add glittery sparkle, Bruce suggests you use a bronze or gold metallic eye shadow on the inner half of your lid. For all your makeup colors, remember that powders last longer than creams.

Use your dark contour shadow on the outer half of your lid and wrap it around to the middle of your bottom rim. This creates the illusion of more and thicker lashes.

For eyelashes that will stay curled, apply a coat of mascara first, then curl with your eyelash curler. Comb to separate lashes before applying a second coat of mascara. When it dries, curl your lashes again.

For lasting dramatic brow color, tissue off your mascara wand. Hold it horizontally and comb your brows up.

SOFT CONTOUR   To contour your cheeks, apply the blusher under your bones for a soft, natural contour. Your cheeks will still be prominent because you've already applied the highlighter above them.

Blush the sides of your neck, collarbone, and between your breasts if your dress is cut low. Blushing around your breasts makes them look fuller, too. Gold powders and bronzers add color excitement to any rich complexion.

Before adding your lip color, first blot with a tissue to remove excess oils that have been activated from the application process. Dust your entire face, including lips, with a sheer layer of your loose powder mixture to doubly set makeup.

LONGEST-LASTING LIP COLOR   Bruce's tip for lasting lip color really works: Begin your lip color by coloring your lips with a matte pencil the same color as the lipstick you are going to use. When your lipstick and gloss disappear, your base color—the pencil—remains for at least an hour longer.

THE RAINPROOF SET   Preserving your hairstyle, especially in bad weather, is your next big challenge. Rain may bring you luck, but it's disaster for maintaining your curls. A top-quality hair spray, which you should always keep handy, is your best guarantee against damp, humid weather. Here is my personally tested tip for a rainproof set.

THE SPRAY SET

Shampoo your hair, following the instructions on page 34. Wet-set your hair. Dry completely under a hooded dryer.

Unwind the rollers and clip the curls in place, using metal clips or bobby pins.

With your hair spray, spritz evenly inside and outside the curls. Let dry completely. Hair should have a light, crispy feeling. Do not get back under the dryer.

Remove the clips or bobby pins and comb and style your hair. When you've completed this step, spray your hair again *very* generously. Let hair dry completely.

You may have to shampoo again the following day to remove the hair spray, but once that special occasion is a success, and you looked gorgeous in spite of the weather, it's worth it!

Fashion and Your Total Beauty Image

• — • — • — • — • — • — • — • — • — • — • — • — • — • — • — • — • — •

It's easy to spot the woman who has taken the time to analyze her body. She's the one who makes heads turn on the street, in a crowded room, on a bus.

Analyzing your body correctly enhances your ability to define your own style. Your beauty image is complete when you make the right fashion statement. Sandra Head, associate fashion editor for *Mademoiselle* magazine, helps you use your most honest friend, the mirror, to take a good, close look at your body.

A familiar theme—organization—helps with co-ordinating your wardrobe. International fashion and beauty consultant, Audrey Smaltz, shares her common-sense shopping and storing tips with you.

YOUR BODY PERSONALITY Fashion editor Sandra Head encourages you to go beyond the fashion limits. First, understand your body personality to determine what particular style is right for you.

Your most important feature is good posture. If you stand or walk incorrectly, no matter how expensive your clothes are, they will always seem slightly off balance.

Double-check to see if your body is aligned properly when you walk. Balance a book on your head, and walk from one side of the room to the other, up and down stairs. You will be aware of where you are throwing your body weight, if you are slouching your shoulders or sticking out your tummy. The only way to keep that book balanced is to walk with your head erect, and extend your legs from your hip sockets, not your waist.

THE NAKED TRUTH   The best way to become acquainted with your body is to analyze it completely nude in front of a full-length mirror. Starting from the top, examine every area of your body for your exact physical proportions. Put on soothing music to help you relax and feel comfortable.

THE SUSPENSION POINT   Shoulders are your suspension point, the bridge that connects and aligns clothes to your body. Shoulders determine how well a garment will fit you.

Take a yardstick and place it horizontally across your shoulders. Lay it in front so that the yardstick is even with the top of your shoulders.

If your shoulders are parallel to the yardstick, they are broad and you rarely will have a fitting problem with your clothes.

If they angle downard, they are sloping and this affects any garment that anchors on your shoulders. Care is necessary in choosing clothes such as halter dresses or tailored blouses.

Shoulders that curve forward are round and change the way your clothing will fit, too. Tops will probably pull in the back and droop in the front. Raglan sleeves are more becoming.

Fleshy arms should be softly draped with clothing, while trim, toned arms can go bare. If your breasts are large, avoid clingy, form-fitting clothes. V-necklines, rather than a high, ruffled collar elongate a short neck.

YOUR WAIST   Your waist is your next important suspension point. It anchors your skirts and pants.

Where is your real waist? Your elbow should meet your waist. If your elbows are higher, you are long-waisted and should avoid separates that call attention to the center part of your body.

If your elbows are lower than your waist, you are short-waisted and should wear overblouses or unbelted dresses to camouflage your waistline and elongate you.

HIPS AND THIGHS   If your hips extend beyond your shoulders, you should avoid pleated or gathered skirts. Check your side profile. A protruding fanny indicates the amount of extra fullness you *don't* need. In general, if you are large, the flow and drape of soft fabrics will give you a more graceful appearance.

Heavy thighs cause pants and jeans to hug snugly. Skirts may be more flattering.

KNEES, CALVES, AND ANKLES Usually, three inches below your knee is where your hemline begins. However, if your calves are very full and round, you may want to slim them by dropping your hemline an inch or two.

Just as hair frames your face, your feet frame your body. They emphasize all your effort in putting yourself together.

Thick ankles are less noticeable if your shoes don't have ankle straps. If your heels are fleshy, pass up slingback shoes. Unattractive toes will be your secret if you avoid open-toe shoes.

SELECTIVE SHOPPING Quality, not quantity, is vital in selecting your fashion wardrobe. You will enjoy more use out of a few classic items. Fashion and beauty consultant Audrey Smaltz suggests that you stick to pure, natural fibers when expanding your wardrobe.

Before you purchase a garment, turn it inside out and check the seams. This gives you a good indication of how well it is made. When buying coats and jackets, make sure you have extra buttons. Most better clothing will have additional ones already sewn in. If they don't, be sure to purchase an extra button or two—just in case.

In order for your clothes to really flatter you, they must fit your body properly. Have altering done *before* you wear something new. Remember that length has little to do with fashion. It's what's flattering on you that's always fashion right.

PLAYING SEPARATELY Separates offer the greatest variety. You can easily vary your outfits when you have separates that are color-coordinated. Buy clothes from season to season that pull together what you already have in your wardrobe. Every once in a while, surprise yourself by purchasing something absolutely frivolous!

Clothing that you receive compliments on should be the ones you wear the most. When traveling, never pack anything you've never worn before. The outfits you feel most comfortable wearing at home are the ones you'll feel comfortable wearing in a new city or country.

Dress-rehearse your clothes to avoid overpacking. When traveling to a warmer climate, have at least one transitional outfit for a surprisingly cool day.

HANGING AROUND   The key to smartly coordinating your clothes is organization. Clothes that you have not worn over a year should be stored or given away. Fashion does repeat itself, but the returning styles always have a new, contemporary twist. Cleaning out your closets seasonally makes room so that you always have space between each garment.

Hang all your skirts together and coordinate by grouping them in light, medium, and dark colors. Follow with blouses, slacks, dresses, jackets, suits.

Keep belts, scarves, shoes together. Plastic bins from dime stores cut down on space and allow you to clearly see everything.

You may want to redesign your closet by adding shelves to suit your particular fashion needs. Organize it so you can always find that hat and pocketbook you need.

If your closet is large, you should have a light inside. Two closets are ideal—one for winter clothing, one for summer.

Wire hangers from the cleaners ruin the shape of your clothes and they should be immediately replaced with plastic, padded, or wooden hangers. Padded hangers preserve the shoulders in your silk blouses, coats, and jackets. Fold, don't hang, jerseys over a nice wide hanger to keep their shape.

SEPARATE DRAWERS   Keep foundations—bras, panties, pantyhose—separately folded. You should always know which drawer has the item you need. A storing trick for hose is to keep them in a large drawstring bag. They are accessible, yet out of your way.

Your wardrobe is not complete without a selection of pantyhose and foundations. Have two or three pairs of hose to coordinate with your basic everyday shoes.

Undergarments should be varied so that you can match whatever you're wearing, or substitute a nude or flesh color to blend in with your clothing. Remember, when you're wearing white, you do not want to wear a white bra which contrasts too much with your dark skin. A flesh color looks neater and more natural.

Wearing the right foundations are vital in order for your clothes to fit properly. Wear underwire bras and comfortable girdles for a smooth line that allows your clothes to fit as well as they were designed.

YOUR COLOR BASE   Now, when you shop, you have a good idea of what is going to be the most flattering garment for you. You can expand your fashion limits, complete your beauty image, with the exciting use of color.

Your mirror is your tool to help you decide where best to apply color. Small shoulders and breasts can take lots of color and prints on top. Large breasts and wide shoulders are de-emphasized with color and prints concentrated on the bottom of your outfit.

Use color dramatically in your clothing. Mix different hues and stretch the fashion limits. As Black women, we automatically think in color. Our base, which is our beautiful skin, gives us a natural attitude, an innate understanding of the use and power of color.

A
Closing
Note

Beauty Is from the Inside Out

This is one of my favorite expressions because it embodies my entire philosophy about true beauty. The great emphasis we place on beautifying our bodies—from luxurious hair and skin treatments to meticulous application of makeup and wearing the right clothing—are only the superficial toppings of making ourselves beautiful.

True beauty radiates from within, has its roots in the heart, mind, and soul, and emanates through you—your face, your smile, and especially, your eyes.

There are many factors that contribute to constructing a solid base of inner beauty. First of all, it extends to establishing a healthy source of spiritual reinforcement from which comes the only true peace and tranquillity. God's love exchanged is so healing for the inner you.

Beyond this, your friends—that circle of people you choose to spend your valued free time with—should be supportive, happy people whom you love and trust and who sincerely love and trust you. Their attitudes and vibrations are part of what your inner self feeds upon. Make them only positive. Negativity can be fatal to the spirit.

Learn to be alone with yourself so that you can become acquainted with who you really are. Spend your time constructively, doing things you like to do, being actively involved in your mental growth and personal development. When you are content to be alone, you learn the secret of enriching your life and the lives of those you love.

And when you deserve applause, don't be timid to be the first one to put your arms around you, hug tightly, and tell yourself you're "wonderful."